Anxiety

James C Ballenger MD
Professor Emeritus
Department of Psychiatry and Behavioral Sciences,
Medical University of South Carolina
Senior Vice President for Scientific Development
Director of Drug Development Division
Comprehensive Neuroscience, Inc.
Charleston, USA

André Tylee MBES, MRCPsych (hon), FRCGP, MD (London)
Professor and Head of Section of Primary
Care Mental Health
Health Services Research Department, Institute of
Psychiatry, London, UK

D1342630

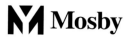 Mosby

MOSBY
An imprint of Elsevier Science Limited.

The
Publisher's
policy is to use
paper manufactured
from sustainable forests

ISBN 0-7234-3313-5

Cataloguing in Publication Data
Catalogue records for this book are available from the US Library of Congress and the British Library.

Note
Medical knowledge is constantly changing. As new information becomes available, changes in treatment, procedures, equipment and the use of drugs become necessary. The editors/authors/contributors and the publishers have taken care to ensure that the information given in this text is accurate and up to date. However, readers are strongly advised to confirm that the information, especially with regard to drug usage, complies with the latest legislation and standards of practice.

Printed by Grafos S.A. Arte sobre papel, Spain.

Contents

Abbreviations

BZ	benzodiazepine
CBT	cognitive behavioural therapy
CCK	cholecystokinin
ECA	Epidemiologic Catchment Area
GABA	gamma aminobuteryic acid
GAD	generalized anxiety disorder
HPA	hypothalamic pituitary axis
LC	locus coeruleus
LSAS	Liebowitz Social Anxiety Scale
MAOI	monoamine oxidase inhibitor
NCS	National Comorbidity Study
NE	norepinephrine
NIH	National Institutes of Health
OCD	obsessive compulsive disorder
PA	panic attacks
PCT	panic control treatment
PD	panic disorder
PET	positron emission tomography
PTSD	post-traumatic stress disorder
RTMS	rapid transcranial magnetic stimulation
SNRI	serotonin-norepinephrine reuptake inhibitor
SSRI	selective serotonin reuptake inhibitors
TCA	tricyclic antidepressant
Y-BOCS	Yale–Brown Obsessive Compulsive Scale

Introduction

The anxiety disorders are the most prevalent psychiatric disorders, affecting over one-quarter of the population and are the most common psychiatric problems presenting to primary care physicians. Over 90% of psychiatric patients present first to primary care with somatic complaints rather than psychological ones.[1] Therefore, knowledge of the features that will distinguish the primary care patient with an anxiety disorder becomes critical, particularly since they are now treatable in many instances by the primary care physician. This short book reviews the five anxiety disorders (panic disorder, generalized anxiety disorder, obsessive compulsive disorder, social anxiety disorder and post-traumatic stress disorder), their clinical features, diagnosis, epidemiology and treatments, hopefully in a format designed for the busy clinician.

Panic Disorder

Description

Panic disorder (PD) is a common and very distressing syndrome of panic attacks (PAs) and worries about those PAs. Such PAs are overwhelming periods of extreme anxiety and physical symptoms that develop suddenly and reach their maximum intensity within 10 minutes (Figure 1). The DSM-IV diagnostic criteria list 13 symptoms for PAs and at least four are required (Table 1). Many of the most common symptoms are physical (e.g. tachycardia, trembling, sweating, etc.) and patients often feel they are dying. Thus, it is not surprising that patients frequently present to general medical settings, emergency rooms and cardiology.

The characteristic time course of a PA is where anxiety levels go from either no or only mild anxiety to maximal, very frightening levels of anxiety very rapidly, over a 10 minute period (Figure 1). After this crescendo, anxiety can fade rapidly. However, many patients describe that they are still anxious and upset for minutes, if not hours later and are typically exhausted afterwards.

The anxiety that patients traditionally develop between PAs has been called anticipatory anxiety because it is largely related

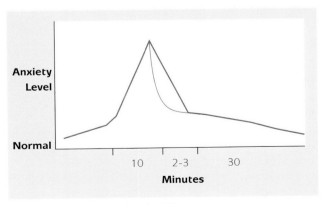

Figure 1. Time course of typical PA.

DSM-IV-TR symptoms of a PA
(1) Palpitations, pounding heart, or accelerated heart rate
(2) Sweating
(3) Trembling or shaking
(4) Sensations of shortness of breath or smothering
(5) Feeling of choking
(6) Chest pain or discomfort
(7) Nausea or abdominal distress
(8) Feeling dizzy, unsteady, light-headed or faint
(9) Derealization (feelings of unreality) or depersonalization (being detached from oneself)
(10) Fear of losing control or going crazy
(11) Fear of dying
(12) Paraesthesiae (numbness or tingling sensations)
(13) Chills or hot flushes

Table 1. DSM-IV-TR symptoms of a PA. Reprinted with permission from the *Diagnostic and Statistical Manual of Mental Disorder Fourth Edition*, Text Revision. Copyright 2000 American Psychatric Association (www.appi.org).

to fears of having another attack or of situations that they fear will elicit another one, e.g. going to the dentist, crossing a bridge, etc.

Diagnosis

The diagnosis of PD (see Table 2)[2] also requires at least a month of concern or worry about:

- having further PAs;
- worry about the implications of the PAs; or
- significant change in behaviour secondary to the attacks.

These PAs cannot be secondary to a medical condition or substance abuse. Although PAs occur in other disorders (e.g. social phobia, post-traumatic stress disorder), it is only in PD that recurrent, unexpected, "out of the blue" attacks occur. For instance, PAs with social phobia occur only in social situations where the person is asked to do something that they are already very afraid of (e.g. eating in front of others, giving a speech). In post-traumatic stress disorder (PTSD) it might be that the patient has no PAs except when confronted with a reminder of their previous trauma. Again, although PAs can occur in

DSM-IV-TR diagnostic criteria for panic disorder without agoraphobia

A. Both (1) and (2)
  (1) recurrent unexpected PAs
  (2) at least one of the attacks has been followed by 1 month (or more) of one (or more) of the following:
    (a) persistent concern about having additional attacks
    (b) worry about the implications of the attack or its consequences (e.g. losing control, having a heart attack, "going crazy")
    (c) a significant change in behaviour related to the attacks

B. Absence of agoraphobia

C. The PAs are not due to the direct physiological effects of a substance (e.g. drug of abuse, a medication) or general medication condition (e.g. hyperthyroidism)

D. The PAs are not better accounted for by another mental disorder, such as social phobia (e.g. occurring on exposure to feared social situations), specific phobia (e.g. on exposure to a specific phobic situation), OCD (e.g. on exposure to dirt in someone with an obsession about contamination), PTSD (e.g. in response to stimuli associated with a severe stressor), or separation anxiety disorder (e.g. in response to being away from home or close relatives)

Table 2. DSM-IV-TR diagnostic criteria for PD without agoraphobia. Reprinted with permission from the *Diagnostic and Statistical Manual of Mental Disorder, Fourth Edition*, Text Revision. Copyright 2000 American Psychatric Association (www.appi.org).

obsessive compulsive disorder (OCD), panic only occurs in OCD when the person is confronted with what they obsessionally fear, for instance an object they believe to be contaminated. The diagnosis of PD is fairly straightforward if the patient has recurrent unexpected PAs, accompanied by changes in their behaviour.

Patients who have fewer than four symptoms in their PAs are said to have "limited symptom attacks." Although these so-called "limited symptom attacks" have fewer symptoms, they can prove equally as distressing and impairing and also respond to treatment in much the same way as full PAs.

The other essential differential diagnostic point is whether or not the patient has developed avoidance of those situations

DSM-IV-TR diagnostic criteria for panic disorder with agoraphobia

A. Both (1) and (2)
  (1) recurrent unexpected PAs
  (2) at least one of the attacks has been followed by 1 month (or more) of one (or more) of the following:
    (a) persistent concern about having additional attacks
    (b) worry about the implications of the attack or its consequences (e.g. losing control, having a heart attack, "going crazy")
    (c) a significant change in behaviour related to the attacks

B. Presence of agoraphobia

C. The PAs are not due to the direct physiological effects of a substance (e.g. drug of abuse, a medication) or general medication condition (e.g. hyperthyroidism)

D. The PAs are not better accounted for by another mental disorder, such as social phobia (e.g. occurring on exposure to feared social situations), specific phobia (e.g. on exposure to a specific phobic situation), OCD (e.g. on exposure to dirt in someone with an obsession about contamination), PTSD (e.g. in response to stimuli associated with a severe stressor), or separation anxiety disorder (e.g. in response to being away from home or close relatives)

Table 3. DSM-IV-TR diagnostic criteria for PD with agoraphobia. Reprinted with permission from the *Diagnostic and Statistical Manual of Mental Disorder, Fourth Edition*, Text Revision. Copyright 2000 American Psychatric Association (www.appi.org).

they fear or where they have previously experienced PAs. This avoidance is called agoraphobia and is the principal predictor of functional impairment. Although the frequency of PAs varies tremendously between individuals, from multiple attacks per day to one every several weeks, avoiding these triggering situations can greatly interfere with function. In the most severe cases (probably 5%), patients completely avoid going out of their home to avoid these terrifying PAs.

It has been estimated from epidemiologic surveys that approximately 50% of individuals who develop recurrent PAs have significant agoraphobic avoidance, with 75% of individuals with PAs having at least some agoraphobic avoidance (see Table 3). [3]

Agoraphobic fears characteristically cluster around certain situations, frequently including travelling by public transportation (buses, trains), motorways, crossing bridges or tunnels, large crowds, or areas where the individual might feel trapped such as elevators, standing in queues, etc. (Table 4). Several of the most frequent ones include fear of going to the supermarket or cinema. However, some patients greatly fear being alone and also experience PAs even at home.

It is important to gauge to what extent patients resist avoiding situations. What situations do they avoid altogether and which ones can they enter? Do they go into the situation anyway and endure it with dread? Do they take a companion along, like their spouse, relative or even a small child? Patients often rationalize that they are taking someone "to help them if they have an attack."

Differential diagnosis

The differential points between PD and the other anxiety disorders are described in Table 5.

Epidemiology

In the National Institute of Mental Health Epidemiologic Catchment Area (ECA) study of 15,000 individuals, the lifetime prevalence of PD was 1.7% (Table 6).[4] In a large

Typical agoraphobic situations

- Queues (e.g. shops, cinemas)
- Supermarkets
- Public transportation (e.g. aeroplanes, trains, buses)
- Enclosed places (e.g. elevators)
- Crowds (e.g. cinemas, ballgames)
- Wide open spaces (e.g. public square)
- Shopping centres
- Bridges or tunnels (because could get "stuck" in traffic)
- Motorways (few exits)
- Situations where "trapped" (e.g. dentist)
- Church

Table 4. Typical agoraphobic situations.

Differential diagnostic features

- PD
  - Recurrent unexpected PAs
  - Avoidance behaviour
- Social phobia (social anxiety disorder)
  - Anxiety only in social situations
  - PAs only when observed performing in public ("embarrassed")
- PTSD
  - Clear history of severe trauma (rape, assault, etc.)
  - PAs only when reminded of trauma
- OCD
  - Rituals and compulsions that cannot be resisted without significant distress
  - PAs only when confronted by obsessional object (e.g. contaminated cloth) or if ritual (e.g. washing) prevented
- Generalized anxiety disorder
  - Worry and anxiety about almost everything
  - Tension, insomnia, headache
  - No PAs

Table 5. Differential diagnostic features.

Epidemiology of PD in community sample

NIMH ECA(1980–1983)

	Prevalence	
	Lifetime	One month
PAs	9.7%	
PD	1.7%	0.5%
Agoraphobia	5.6%	

National Comorbidity Study (NCS) (1990–1992)

	Prevalence	
	Lifetime	One month
PAs	15.6%	
PD	3.5%	1.5%
Agoraphobia	6.7%	

Table 6. Epidemiology of PD in community samples.

follow-up study, the National Comorbidity Study (NCS), the lifetime prevalence was estimated at 3.5%. The lifetime prevalence for agoraphobia was 5.6% in the ECA study and 6.7% in the NCS.[5]

It is important to recognize the high frequency of PAs in the population. In the ECA study, 9.7% of the population had PAs sometime in their lifetime. The NCS study documented this rate at 15.6%. Other data suggest that 10% of the population have a PA yearly. Differences between these figures and figures for the diagnosis of PD itself relate to the fact that some people have one or two PAs but do not develop recurrent unexpected PAs, secondary anxiety or changes in their behaviour. Apparently, it is recurrent severe PAs that lead people to become ill and to develop anticipatory anxiety, fears of being in certain situations and functional difficulty because of these fears.

PD is generally three times more common in women and is also a young person's illness, with a peak incidence in the third decade, although frequently patients report that they have had anxiety all their lives. Typically, patients vividly report their first PA and often are able to describe a situation of increased stress in their life at that time.

Pathogenesis

Most of the hypotheses about the aetiology of PD (and the other anxiety disorders) centre on putative neurotransmitter abnormalities, principally norepinephrine (NE), serotonin and gamma-amino buteryic acid (GABA). Evidence for the involvement of one or more of these neurotransmitter systems in PD comes from a series of animal, laboratory and neurobiological studies. However, it is the indirect evidence from medications that have been observed to work in PD, and their effect on these neurotransmitters, that has largely supported these theories.

Norepinephrine

The NE neurons in the brain primarily originate in a mid-brain nucleus, the locus coeruleus (LC), and project to limbic areas, such as the amygdala, as well as to cortical areas, most particularly the frontal lobe (Figure 2). Animal studies suggest

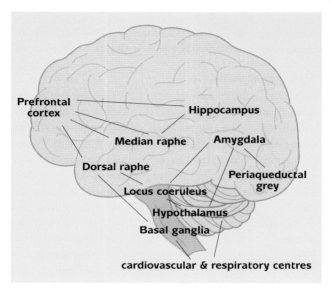

Figure 2. Brain anxiety circuit.

that stimulation of the LC results in severe anxiety, suggesting that this pathway is critical for PD. Because the two inhibitor neurotransmitters (serotonin and GABA) and the principal excitatory neurons (glutamate) also impinge on the NE neuron and all effective medications decrease the firing rate of the LC, this system has been thought to be involved in PD. In addition to the theory that NE is simply increased in PD, data also suggest that a disregulation of the NE system may be critical.[6]

Serotonin
The serotonin system has been postulated to be involved in multiple psychiatric syndromes, primarily because of the success of the selective serotonin reuptake inhibitors (SSRIs) in treating both depression and all five of the anxiety disorders. There are two sets of serotonin nuclei: the dorsal raphe, which primarily projects to the cerebral cortex; and the median raphe, which projects to limbic structures including the hippocampus. A series of studies suggest that both increased serotonin and decreased serotonin reduce anxiety levels. Recent research

demonstrates that treatment with the SSRI fluoxetine actually reduces NE volatility levels to the normal range,[7] which could potentially explain these disparate findings.

Neuroanatomy

There is now sufficient evidence to suggest that a relatively specific anatomical circuit in the brain underlies fear and anxiety. This circuit includes the amygdala, hippocampus, prefrontal cortex, periaqueductal grey and the LC (Figure 2).[8] These reciprocally connected areas appear to be involved in most of the behavioural responses of fear, freezing and escape. Most interestingly for PD, these areas are also intimately connected to structures that seem to control the multiple physical symptoms accompanying panic, including increased heart rate (vagus), increased respiration (nucleus parabrachialis) and increased levels of cortisol (via hypothalamus, LC and tegmentum).

Physical examination

Physical examination in PD is generally normal, although increases in pulse rate and labile hypertension can be observed.

Laboratories

Routine CBC, electrolytes, calcium and thyroid function tests are indicated for most patients (Table 7). There are no characteristic laboratory abnormalities, although the chronic overbreathing leads to respiratory alkalosis. More elaborate testing should be reserved for specific issues suggested by the history and physical examination.

Course

Once PD becomes established, it is generally a chronic condition that often worsens over time, especially with increases in avoidance. Exacerbations are common in times of stress.

Functional impairment

Surprisingly, the physical and social impairment of PD is often worse than that found in patients with major depression or other chronic conditions.

Suggested laboratory studies in PD
• CBC • Electrolytes • Calcium • Thyroid • Urine screen for drugs • Liver function tests (if cryptic alcohol abuse suspected) • Other tests suggested by history and physical examination • ECG (over age 40)

Table 7. Suggested laboratory studies in PD.

Presentation in primary care

Anxiety has been reported to be the most common psychiatric problem seen in primary care,[9] with PD occurring in as many as 13% of primary care patients.[10] Unfortunately in the large worldwide WHO Primary Care Study, over one-half of panic patients were undiagnosed.[11]

It is probably the primarily somatic presentation of the PD patient, coupled with their strong insistence that something is physically wrong with them that leads to such high rates of misdiagnosis. Patients usually present in a very frightened state with a conviction that there is a physical cause for their difficulties, generally centring around the organ of their principal physical symptoms. Therefore, those with chest pain, tachycardia and palpitations, frequently present to a cardiologist, whilst those with gastrointestinal symptoms suggestive of irritable bowel syndrome present to a gastroenterologist. PD patients are five to eight times more likely to be high utilizers of medical services,[12] leading to marked increases in overall health care costs.[13]

Comorbidity

As with all the anxiety disorders, being comorbid with other anxiety, depressive or substance abuse disorders is quite common. Generalized anxiety disorder (GAD), social phobia (up to one-third) and PTSD are commonly seen with PD.

Certainly one of the most common comorbid conditions is depression and two out of three PD patients develop depression at some time in their lifetime. This frequently occurs after years of difficulties with PD, although depression can occur both prior to, and at the same time as, PD.

Comorbidity with any of these disorders, particularly depression, certainly complicates treatment and increases the distress, functional impairment and suicide risk. Alcohol abuse and dependence frequently occur, often as individuals try to manage their anxiety by drinking.

Treatment

Treatment of PD typically involves the use of new panic medications and cognitive behavioural therapy (CBT), which exposes patients to phobic situations or at least supportive psychotherapy. Guidelines have been promulgated by the National Institutes of Health (NIH) in a consensus meeting in 1992 and, more recently, by the International Consensus Group for Depression and Anxiety[14] and the American Psychiatric Association Practice Guidelines.[15]

Pharmacotherapy

At this point in time, the SSRIs have become the treatment of choice for not only depression but all five of the anxiety disorders. A series of studies with the SSRIs paroxetine (40–60 mg/day),[16] sertraline (50–200 mg/day),[17] fluoxetine (20–60 mg/day),[18] fluvoxamine (150–300 mg/day)[19] and citalopram (20–40 mg/day),[20] as well as meta-analyses, all suggest that SSRIs are more effective than the tricyclics or alprazolam.[21] Many of these well-controlled trials are short-term studies, but recent long-term studies also support their long-term use and most clinicians treat patients for 12–24 months.

With all antidepressant medications, the panic patient should begin with low doses (2.5–5 mg fluoxetine, 5–10 mg paroxetine) with gradually increasing doses to avoid the characteristic activating side-effects, often called the "jitteriness syndrome". Patients often develop increases in anxiety, tremor

SSRIs in PD	
Positives:	• Little weight gain • Treat common comorbid disorders (depression, social phobia, OCD, GAD, PTSD) • No dry mouth, constipation, blurred vision (anticholinergic side-effects) • No cardiovascular side-effects (dizziness, conduction effects) • Non-addictive • No interaction with alcohol • Safe in overdose
Negative:	• Sexual side-effects and nausea

Table 8. SSRIs in PD.

and insomnia if treatment is begun at the higher doses (used for the treatment of depression) and discontinue treatment because of their fears.

The SSRIs have become the treatment of choice because they are at least as effective as any other treatments and are markedly better tolerated (see Table 8 for advantages).

Benzodiazepines

Alprazolam was the first benzodiazepine (BZ) shown to be effective in short-term treatment of PD with or without agoraphobia.[22] Unlike antidepressant treatment of PD, in which 3–6 weeks or longer is required to see significant beneficial effects, BZs often produce effects within the first week. Studies have demonstrated that the average daily dose of alprazolam is 1–10 mg/day (given tid or qid), with an average of 5.7 mg/day in the largest trial.[22] In a large, multinational trial, alprazolam and imipramine were equally effective but alprazolam was more rapidly effective.

Another commonly utilized BZ is clonazepam, effective at doses approximately half that of alprazolam (e.g. 2.5 mg/day). Because of its longer half-life, clonazepam can be given only twice daily. Clinical lore suggests that there is less inter-dose rebound anxiety with clonazepam (i.e. less return of anxiety when the blood levels fall between doses).[23] Clonazepam's longer half-life also makes it more suitable for prn use in PD, or with varying doses from day to day, because fewer withdrawal symptoms appear to occur than with alprazolam.

Combining of BZs with antidepressants

BZs are very frequently combined with antidepressants, with the clinical expectation that BZs will work rapidly and can be tapered later on. Despite how common this practice is, it is not well supported by controlled trials, one of which found that the combination was actually less effective.[24]

Long-term use of BZs

Use of BZs, especially long-term, has been associated with multiple concerns and fears that tolerance will develop, that they will be abused or that discontinuation will be very difficult, particularly with high potency BZs (alprazolam, clonazepam). The widely held negative opinion of BZs is not supported by the evidence.[25] Tolerance is not observed nor is abuse of BZs a significant issue in patients with PD. It has been found that very few patients escalate their dose, and, in fact, the larger clinical problem is actually getting patients to take sufficient doses to treat their panic anxiety. The main issues with BZs are avoiding prescribing BZs to patients who abuse other substances and the lack of understanding of the importance of tapering the dosage when discontinuing treatment (see below).

BZ discontinuation

Evidence suggests that if patients are informed and educated about the discontinuation process and receive slowly tapered doses then they are usually able to discontinue BZs without incident.[26] Good clinical practice requires that the patient and his/her family are well educated about the effects of discontinuing treatment and can have all their questions answered about symptoms that can occur during the discontinuation phase.

Probably because of increased sensitivity to symptoms, PD patients should be gradually withdrawn from all medicines, particularly BZs. A taper period lasting between 2 and 4 months, and perhaps even 6 months is strongly recommended. CBT has been found to be helpful for some PD patients who are discontinuing BZs.[27]

Positives and negatives aspects of BZs

The BZs have several advantages, principally that they are rapidly effective, well tolerated, reduce anticipatory anxiety and are safe in overdose (Table 9). The main disadvantages include their interaction with alcohol and the occurrence of short-term memory problems in some individuals. In addition, they can be abused and withdrawal symptoms can occur if they are not properly tapered. Perhaps the most significant drawback in the use of BZs is that they fail to block the emergence of depression.[28] This is a major issue since two out of three PD patients will be become depressed in their lifetime, and approximately one-third will become depressed every 2 years.

Tricyclic antidepressants

Imipramine was one of the first antidepressants shown to work in PD. More recently, clomipramine has been shown to be even more effective than imipramine in doses of 150–200 mg/day, and occasionally effective even at very low doses (25 mg/day). However, tricyclic antidepressants (TCAs), even clomipramine,

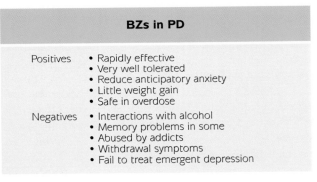

	BZs in PD	
Positives	• Rapidly effective • Very well tolerated • Reduce anticipatory anxiety • Little weight gain • Safe in overdose	
Negatives	• Interactions with alcohol • Memory problems in some • Abused by addicts • Withdrawal symptoms • Fail to treat emergent depression	

Table 9. BZs in PD.

Tricyclics in PD

Positives	• Effective
	• Are antidepressants
	• Non-abused
Negatives	• Significant weight gain
	• "Jitteriness" syndrome problematic
	• Dry mouth, constipation, blurred vision (anticholinergic)
	• Cardiovascular effects (problematic hypotension, increased pulse rate, conduction delays)
	• Can be lethal in overdose

Table 10. Tricyclics in PD.

Other medications in PD

Traditional (irreversible) MAOI	
Phenelzine	45–90 mg/d (mean doses 55–75 mg/d)
Tranylcypromine	10–40 mg/d
Reversible MAO-A inhibitors	
Brofaromine	50–105 mg/d (mean dose 107.2 mg/d)
Buspirone	30–60 mg/d (mean 55 mg/d)

Table 11. Other medications in PD.

are rarely used at this point because of their significant side-effects (Table 10). The high incidence of jitteriness leading to drop outs and their lethality in overdoses, have led the TCAs to be used only infrequently.

Monoamine oxidase inhibitors

The monoamine oxidase inhibitors (MAOIs) (Table 11) are also not commonly used, although the irreversible MAOIs phenelzine and tranylcypromine are quite effective[29] and may be even more effective than other medications.[28,29] MAOIs have all of the negative side-effects of the TCAs, but also require the special restriction of tyramine in the diet and have a risk of hypertensive crisis.

The reversible MAOIs (RIMAs) like brofaramine and meclobamide have been promising in early tests. However, neither is available in the United States and meclobamide is available only in Europe, Canada and South America.

Other antidepressants
Nefazodone and venlafaxine have both been studied in other trials and shown to be effective.[30]

Other agents
The anti-epileptic valproic acid has been reported to have some efficacy in PD, as has gabapentin, whereas carbamazepine appears not to be effective.

Buspirone
The 5-HT-$_{1A}$ receptor agonist buspirone, although widely utilized in generalized anxiety, does not appear to be effective in the treatment of PD. Beta-blockers, are widely used but the recent conclusion of an international panel was that they should not be utilized as a primary treatment for PD.[31]

Long-term treatment
Most PD patients who have a syndrome severe enough to require treatment are generally treated for 12–24 months before consideration is given to tapering and decreasing medications to see if they are still necessary. The SSRIs have emerged as the main treatment for PD largely because they are so well tolerated.

Issues of maintenance therapy
With long-term treatment, the principal side-effect of SSRIs, namely increasing sexual dysfunction, occurs in or with increasing frequency. Although other antidepressants and BZs can also cause sexual dysfunction, the SSRIs are the most common. Frequent problems include delayed orgasm in both males and females, as well as reduced libido and erectile dysfunction in males. The most common strategies to deal

with this include educating the patient, allowing time to pass, reducing doses or the use of other medicines to try to block these side-effects. Other medicines that have been shown to be helpful include amantadine (50–100 mg), bupropion (100–200 mg), buspirone (30–60 mg) or bethanacol (10–20 mg) taken before intercourse. A popular clinical strategy at this point is the use of sildenafil. Other strategies include 1 or 2 day drug holidays or switching to another medication, such as nefazodone or potentially bupropion, although it is uncertain how effective it is in PD.

Treatment during pregnancy

Because PD occurs in such high frequency in young women another common issue is the use of medication during or after pregnancy. While some women greatly improve in terms of their PD during pregnancy, others do not change or actually worsen. Antidepressants have not been shown to cause any serious adverse effects on the pregnancy or the outcome of pregnancy.[32] A recent review concluded that the risk of nontreatment is thought to be greater than treatment.

Current recommendations are that medications should be avoided if possible and certainly during the first trimester, using CBT or other psychotherapies instead. Certainly the use of BZs can lead to physiological dependence and therefore withdrawal in a newborn, so it should not be used if possible. These decisions should be made in collaboration with the psychiatrist, patient and obstetrician.

In breastfeeding women with PD, the more highly protein-bound medicines, paroxetine, sertraline and fluoxetine, should be utilized.[33]

Reasons for poor response

Table 12 lists the common reasons for inadequate response to medications.

Psychosocial treatment

There are multiple empirically validated psychotherapies for PD, but few patients actually receive them at this point in time,[34]

Factors to consider if response to treatment inadequate

- Dose too low
- Treatment too short (12–16 weeks needed)
- Poor compliance
- Unrecognized comorbid condition (e.g. depression, OCD, PTSD, social phobia)
- Substance abuse/withdrawal
- Failure to perform exposure aspects of treatment
- Unrecognized medical disorder
- Need individual or couple psychotherapy
- Severe stress in life

Table 12. Factors to consider if response to treatment inadequate.

which is primarily related to the lack of trained therapists, especially in primary care. This is one of the principal reasons for specialist referral, i.e. if the patient requires psychotherapy, either from preference or a failure to respond adequately to pharmacotherapy.

Cognitive behavioural therapy

An essential element of psychotherapeutic treatment of PD, and particularly agoraphobia, involves re-exposure to the phobic situation. During exposure treatments, patients are generally gradually exposed to the situations they fear and are avoiding. Exposure can occur either in imagery or in actual fact and is often paired with relaxation techniques. Exposure can be accomplished either by the patient alone, with a spouse, or often with recovered phobics who accompany the patient as part of a support group. There is some evidence that flooding techniques, in which a patient has multiple exposure experiences over a short period of time, may be more effective, although it is understandably associated with a high drop out rate. While exposure appears to be essential to any effective psychotherapy of agoraphobia, some exposure techniques are associated with a significant drop out rate. It was this that led to the development of various CBTs.

Panic control treatment

Certainly, the best studied and well known of the CBT treatments for panic is known as panic control treatment (PCT).[35] This involves, as do most of the CBTs, basic education about the nature of panic and the models utilized to understand it. It also involves a cognitive therapy component of identifying and attempting to correct "maladaptive thoughts" about anxiety, learning certain techniques to reduce acute anxiety symptoms, and gradual exposure to bodily sensations (interoceptive exposure) similar to symptoms of PAs (e.g. dizziness, tachycardia). Multiple studies have demonstrated the effectiveness of this treatment with response rates comparable or better than medication treatments.

Practical forms of CBT

Due to the relative unavailability of trained PCT therapists, other forms have been explored, including the use of the telephone or use of self-study modules with a manual, such as the workbook *Mastery of Your Anxiety and Panic*.[36] Others have explored using other self-help books, computer programs and interactive voice-response, or virtual reality systems. All of these have shown promising results, and they offer practical help for the interested primary care physician.

Combination of psychotherapy and pharmacotherapy

Although most clinicians believe a combination of CBT and pharmacotherapy would be more effective, most studies do not in fact find the combination superior to either treatment alone.[37]

However, clinical evidence and some research support the addition of exposure therapy to pharmacotherapy in patients with agoraphobic avoidance. This can be accomplished by the relatively simple instructions to gradually approach previously feared situations, moving steadily over time from the lowest feared situation to the most feared. In addition, interested patients might find helpful assistance in the books and manuals mentioned above.

Relapse

When medications are discontinued or even tapered, a number of patients relapse back into their original PD syndrome. Until recently, this percentage was thought to be as high as 60–90%, although recent studies suggest it may be significantly lower, in the 15–35% range. There is some suggestion that longer treatment (12–24 months) may result in lower relapse rates when medications are discontinued.

Indications for specialist referral

Treatment of the average patient with PD can certainly begin in primary care. Education of the patient through direct education as well as reading articles and books about PD, followed by the initiation of low dose medications, raised gradually, can result in substantial improvement in many patients. Specialist involvement (Table 13) is often indicated to focus the patient's treatment and to provide reassurance, as well as to provide specialized treatments or support groups.

Reasons for specialist referral

- Confirmation of diagnosis (for patient and MD)
- Reassurance of patient to increase motivation for recommended treatments
- Need psychotherapy, support or exposure therapy
- Severe symptomatology
- Failure to improve (after 3 months)
- Comorbidity, e.g. alcoholism, OCD, social phobia
- Recommendation: one consultation at beginning and another 3–6 months later

Table 13. Reasons for specialist referral.

Generalized Anxiety Disorder

Introduction

Generalized Anxiety Disorder (GAD) is the anxiety disorder that we have learned the most about in recent years, particularly in terms of treatment. More accurate diagnosis and treatment in primary care is critical because this disorder is most often seen in the general medical setting. It is usually comorbid with other conditions and a recent study suggested that it complicates perhaps as many as half of all psychiatric and medical conditions.[38]

GAD was first recognized diagnostically in the DSM-III in 1980. It was then considered a wastebasket term because it did not have specific defining features, e.g. phobias, obsessions, PAs. Patients with this disorder have persistent, if not continuous, increased anxiety of a diffuse nature accompanied by autonomic symptoms, particularly somatic tension, vigilance and worry. Subsequent revisions of the diagnostic criteria culminated in the DSM-IV published in 1994 (Table 14). We now consider that GAD involves characteristic excessive and uncontrolled worrying, plus anxiety and somatic symptoms of muscle tension, sleep disturbance, fatigue, irritability, restlessness and difficulty concentrating (see Tables 14 and 15). The most important diagnostic change was the emphasis on chronic, uncontrollable worry lasting for 6 months, together with the physical symptoms that have been recognized all along to accompany this disorder.

Clinical picture

Most patients present to medical physicians not with complaints of uncontrolled worry but with one of the numerous physical symptoms of GAD. These traditionally include muscular tension with neck and back pain and headache, symptoms of feeling restless or keyed up and insomnia. There is a high prevalence of GAD in patients with unexplained somatic symptoms[39] and in patients with irritable bowel syndrome, hypertension, heart disease and diabetes.[40] On questioning, GAD patients do admit that they worry about many areas, essentially all areas of their life including health, finances, family, work, etc. (see Table 16). What

---

Simplified DSM-IV diagnostic criteria for GAD

A. Excessive anxiety and worry (apprehensive expectation), occurring more days than not for at least 6 months, about a number of events or activities

B. The person finds it difficult to control the worry

C. The anxiety and worry are associated with three or more of the following six symptoms:
  (1) Restlessness or feeling keyed up or on edge
  (2) Being easily fatigued
  (3) Difficulty concentrating or mind going blank
  (4) Irritability
  (5) Muscle tension
  (6) Sleep disturbance

D. The focus of the anxiety and worry is not confined to features of another axis I disorder

E. Symptoms cause clinically significant distress or impairment in social, occupational or other important areas of functioning

F. The disturbance is not due to the direct physiological effects of a substance or a general medical condition, and does not occur exclusively during a mood disorder, psychotic disorder or pervasive developmental disorder

Table 14. Simplified DSM-IV diagnostic criteria for GAD. Adapted with permission from the American Psychiatric Association (www.appi.org); copyright 1994.

Physical symptoms of GAD

- Insomnia (principally difficulty falling asleep although also restless sleep)
- Muscle tension (neck tightness, back pain)
- Headache
- Fatigue
- Restlessness
- Irritability

Table 15. Physical symptoms of GAD.

Worries in GAD
Minor hassles (daily issues, time problems, etc.) Family Money Health Work School Interpersonal relationships *Worry is uncontrollable even if thought to be unrealistic

Table 16. Worries in GAD.

distinguishes the worrying of GAD subjects is that it can occupy the majority of the day, they cannot control it or "stop worrying," even though they recognize it is about quite minor matters.

Course

Unlike many of the other anxiety disorders that begin in childhood, GAD tends to begin in the early 20s and peak in the third decade, with a chronic course of fluctuating severity, with symptoms increasing with periods of stress. Without treatment few patients recover.

Differential diagnosis

The principal difficulty in the differential diagnosis of GAD is that the majority of GAD patients also have an additional diagnosis, with social phobia and dysthymia being the most common (Table 17). In the primary care setting, 89% of GAD patients met criteria for an additional comorbid psychiatric disorder.[41]

The differential with depression is the most difficult, particularly mild depression, with GAD-type anxiety commonly preceding or following depression or co-existing with depression. This differential is primarily based on how severe the depressive symptoms are and the characteristic depressive symptoms of hopelessness, anhedonia and suicidal thoughts.

GAD is differentiated from the other anxiety disorders that also have diffuse anxiety by the presence or absence of the

Common comorbid conditions in GAD
• Depression or dysthymia • Substance abuse, especially alcoholism • Other anxiety disorders, e.g. social anxiety disorder and PD • Medical conditions (at least one-third of cases)

Table 17. Common comorbid conditions in GAD.

characteristic features of the other anxiety disorders, e.g. PAs in PD, obsessions in OCD, etc. Probably one of the most difficult differentials is with alcoholism. The majority of alcoholic patients report anxiety and use of alcohol to self mediate; however, alcoholism and alcohol withdrawal can themselves cause anxiety and the diagnosis of GAD needs to be made after the patient has been alcohol-free for at least 3–6 weeks.

Epidemiology

An international WHO trial found an 8% prevalence in primary care, making it the second most common disorder, behind depression.[42,43] Despite changing criteria over the past 20 years, studies in the US, Europe and Asia have suggested a lifetime rate of between 3.4% and 10.5%.

The largest recent study[44] again observed a 1 year prevalence rate of 3.1% and lifetime rate of 5.1%. It has been found that 90% of the lifetime GAD patients had at least one other DSM disorder (most commonly depression and PD). Two-thirds of patients with current GAD had another disorder, again depression, social anxiety disorder and PD being the most common. GAD is probably the most common anxiety disorder in the elderly, with a prevalence of almost 20%.[45]

Despite the fact that GAD peaks after the age of 18, over-anxious disorder is actually the most common psychiatric problem in children, occurring in 3.6–5.9% of children. In the largest study, the 3 month prevalence was 4.4%, twice as common in girls, and increasing in prevalence from age 8–16 years.[46]

Genetics

Some studies suggest that GAD has a genetic or at least a familial cause. Approximately 20% of first degree relatives also have the disorder (five to six times higher than expected) and in twin studies, heritability among female twins was 30%.[47] It may be that GAD is inherited only in those who also inherit a linked gene for depression,[48] perhaps explaining the almost two-thirds comorbidity of these two disorders.

Neuroimaging

The amygdala appears to be involved in the brain anxiety response and multiple positron emission tomography (PET) and functional magnetic resonance imaging studies support involvement of the amygdala and related circuits in GAD and other anxiety disorders. PET scan results suggest increases in metabolism in the right posterior temporal lobe, left inferior frontal lobes, right precentral frontal areas, as well as in the cerebellum and occipital lobes.[49] Increases in basal ganglia and right parietal areas and decreases in right temporal and occipital lobes during vigilance tasks were not normalized with BZs. This suggests that basal ganglia, occipital, temporal and perhaps frontal lobes are involved in abnormal circuitry that contributes to the chronic worrying pattern.

Neurotransmitters

Norepinephrine

The LC system, which is responsible for most of the brain NE activity, has long been known to be involved with vigilance.[50] Some studies, although inconsistent, suggest that GAD is associated with chronic over-secretion of NE[51], which is consistent with the finding that a tricyclic such as imipramine is effective in the treatment of GAD (Table 18).

Serotonin

Certainly the excellent therapeutic results of the SSRIs in GAD (see below) suggest that serotonin is involved in the aetiology of GAD. Studies do suggest involvement of multiple serotonin receptor subtypes 5-HT$_{1A}$, 5-HT$_{2A}$, 5-HT$_{2C}$ and 5-HT$_3$.[52] The 5-HT$_{1A}$ partial agonist buspirone has been shown to be effective in GAD.

Gamma-amino buteryic acid

GABA is the principal inhibitory neurotransmitter in the brain. This, coupled with the clear efficacy of the BZs that interact with the $GABA_A$ receptor complex, implicates GABA receptors in the aetiology of GAD. Some evidence suggests that there are fewer BZ receptor sites that increase with BZ treatment.[53] Tihonen and colleagues report results consistent with decreased BZ receptors in the left temporal lobe in GAD.[54]

Cholecystokinin

Animal, and some human, studies suggest that brain cholecystokinin $(CCK)_B$ receptors may be involved in anxiety[55] but studies with CCK antagonists have been disappointing to date.[56]

Psychosocial factors

Most experts believe that patients' thinking patterns play a significant role in maintaining, if not causing, GAD. Most researchers agree that dysfunctional worries are the core descriptive and perhaps aetiologic feature of GAD and perhaps a key to treatment as well. The GAD patient tends to have automatic anxiety thoughts that prevent them from involving themselves in new situations and learning that their worries are unrealistic. This avoidance leads to chronic over-estimation of the potential dangerousness or probability for failure. Treatment seeks to reverse this pathological thinking and escape

---

Neurochemical abnormalities postulated in GAD

NE
- Especially alpha-2 presynaptic receptor

Serotonin
- Receptor $5\text{-}HT_{1A}$ subtypes $5\text{-}HT_{2C}$, $5\text{-}HT_{2A}$, $5\text{-}HT_{1A}$

GABA
- $GABA_A$

CCK
- CCK_A, CCK_B, CCK_4, CCK_8

Table 18. Neurochemical abnormalities postulated in GAD

behaviour. CBT leads to challenge of these worry/ruminations and has proved to be highly effective (see below).

Lifestyle issues

Certainly caffeine, cigarettes and alcohol should be eliminated to reduce anxiety. Some patients find that physical exercise and yoga reduce their anxiety levels (Table 19).

Pharmacotherapy

Benzodiazepines

Historically, the greatest amount of research and clinical experience in treating GAD has been with BZs. However, their use is highly controversial in some countries, especially the UK and in many primary care settings. However, BZs have been popular because of their clear efficacy, rapid onset, low side-effects and increase in safety over previously available treatments including barbiturates.[57] Many clinicians, and the public, worry about the abuse potential of BZs, although abuse is rare in clinical settings and it is primarily associated with drug abusing individuals. This has lead some experts to suggest that BZs should only be used for periods of less than 4 weeks at low doses.[58] Other authorities have suggested that concerns about the risk of dependence and abuse are so low, and efficacy of BZs so high, that these worries and limitation of use are not justified.[59] Actually a much larger clinical issue is the discontinuation of BZs, particularly after long-term use, high doses or high potency BZs, such as alprazolam and clonazepam, when tapered too rapidly.[60] Predictors of withdrawal severity include

Lifestyle issues

Reduce caffeine and nicotine consumption
Eliminate using alcohol to reduce or control anxiety
Exercise regularly
Try yoga or meditation
Reduce stress where possible

Table 19. Lifestyle issues.

residual levels of anxiety and depression and personality traits such as dependency.

Most clinicians and experts believe that the anxiety present after the appropriate and gradual taper of BZs is actually the return of the basic anxiety problem and this is particularly true with chronic conditions such as GAD.[61]

Despite the controversy there are several unequivocal problems with BZs, including memory and cognitive problems as well as the occasional increases in hostility.[60] The emergence of depression in patients taking BZs also occurs[28] and this suggests that they have no prophylactic value to prevent the very frequent comorbidity with depression. This may be the main reason to suggest that BZs are not currently appropriate for the primary treatment of GAD now that SSRIs have been shown to be at least as effective. The difficulties in tapering, memory disturbances and the actual limited response of many patients treated with BZs has relegated them to primarily adjunctive use in the treatment of GAD and other anxiety disorders.

Many clinicians find that the as needed (prn) use of clonazepam is useful, particularly during periods of increased stress. Although the high potency of alprazolam (high anxiolysis versus low sedation) is occasionally needed, the longer half-life of clonazepam allows greater ease in prn use (see Table 20).

Buspirone

The partial $5-HT_{1A}$ receptor agonist buspirone has been shown to be effective in several trials[62] and has been utilized widely in

BZs in GAD	
Suggested use:	prn or as augmenting agents to antidepressants
Clonazepam:	0.25–0.5 mg bid to qid
Alprazolam:	0.25–0.5 tid (must be tapered slowly often over 4 weeks or longer)

Table 20. BZs in GAD.

the place of the BZs. It is the lack of negative cognitive effects and lack of alcohol potentiation that has led to the popularity of buspirone over the BZs, coupled with its lack of withdrawal symptomatology.[63] Despite its popularity as a "non-BZ," its late onset (2 weeks), multiple negative trials and widespread patient and clinician belief that these agents are less effective[64] have led to limitation of its use. Evolving evidence suggests that it may actually be more useful in patients with depression.[65]

The recent demonstration of SSRIs as effective agents in GAD but without the negative side-effects associated with the BZs or buspirone has put the long-term use of 5-HT$_{1A}$ agonists like buspirone in question.

Hydroxyzine

The histamine (H1) receptor antagonist hydroxyzine is thought to be effective in GAD and has gained widespread use in Europe. Studies are limited but suggest onset of efficacy within the first week and is comparable to at least lorazepam.[66] Interestingly, efficacy has been observed to continue even after abrupt discontinuation. Future studies are clearly warranted to determine the place of hydroxyzine in the treatment of GAD.

Antidepressants

Although labelled as antidepressants, this broad class of medications have been consistently shown to be effective in treating not only the anxiety of depressed patients, but also more recently the anxiety of GAD and the other anxiety disorders. In fact, recent studies suggest that antidepressants over 6–8 weeks are more effective than BZs in treating GAD, although the onset of action of BZs is faster.[67] Early studies with even low doses of the TCA imipramine (mean 91 mg/day) demonstrated efficacy over alprazolam. Interestingly, imipramine demonstrated more efficacy against cognitive symptoms (e.g. negative thoughts, worry, symptoms, etc.), with some suggestion that somatic measures (e.g. cardiovascular, sleep) responded better to the BZ alprazolam. Imipramine appeared to be more effective in reducing anticipatory worry and depressive symptoms, leading to the current recommendations that antidepressants would be better treatments than BZs for chronic worry, difficulties with interpersonal relationships and frequent depression in GAD.

In a study comparing imipramine (mean 143 mg/day) and trazodone (255 mg/day) to diazepam (26 mg/day), the highest response rates (73% and 69%) were seen with imipramine and trazodone with 47% responding to diazepam. Again, the antidepressants were more effective against psychic symptoms, but in this trial both the antidepressants and BZ were more effective than placebo against the somatic symptoms of GAD.

Venlafaxine

These early studies with imipramine and trazodone lead to the first large-scale trials with the antidepressant venlafaxine, an SNRI (serotonin-NE reuptake inhibitor). After promising short trials comparing venlafaxine to placebo, and other trials with buspirone to diazepam, venlafaxine became the first antidepressant to receive FDA approval in the US for treatment of GAD. Importantly, venlafaxine was shown to be effective against both the psychic and somatic symptoms of GAD.

In the comparison with buspirone, venlafaxine was as least as effective, if not more. In the first long-term study of an antidepressant in GAD, venlafaxine XR 75–225 mg/day maintained its efficacy over a 28-week period, leading to even greater improvement over time (see below).

SSRIs

In the first study of an SSRI (paroxetine 20 mg/day) compared to imipramine and a BZ (2-chlordesmethyldiazepam 3–6 mg/day) in GAD, both antidepressants were more effective than the BZ (paroxetine at week 4 and imipramine at week 8). Again the antidepressants were more effective in resolving the psychic symptoms and the BZ was more effective in resolving the somatic symptoms.

Not surprisingly, patients on imipramine had more anticholinergic side-effects (dry mouth and constipation) than the SSRI or BZ. Again as expected, although generally better tolerated, paroxetine had a higher incidence of nausea, but drop out rates were lowest for paroxetine.

The first large, multi-centre trial with an SSRI was a fixed dose study comparing 20–40 mg/day paroxetine (n = 566). Both doses were highly effective with no observable difference between the two doses.[68] Two 8-week flexible dose studies with paroxetine (20–50 mg/day) again also demonstrated it to be an effective and well-tolerated treatment for GAD.[69,70] In these studies, efficacy against the main symptoms of GAD, anxiety and tension, were observed by the first and third weeks of treatment, respectively. A recent long-term 6-month study of GAD demonstrated fewer relapses with continued paroxetine (11%) than with placebo (40%).

Other SSRIs

Although no trials with citalopram, fluvoxamine, fluoxetine or sertraline have yet been published, clinical experience suggests they may be effective.

Dose

If imipramine were to be utilized in the treatment of GAD, effective responses have been observed at lower doses than utilized in the treatment of depression, e.g. 100 mg/day. Dose finding trials with venlafaxine were not definitive but suggest 75 and 150 mg/day of venlafaxine XR are both effective. Trials with paroxetine again suggest that 20 and 40 mg/day are equally effective (Table 21). Although patients can begin on 20 mg of paroxetine or 75 mg of venlafaxine, many clinicians begin at even lower doses (e.g. 10 mg paroxetine and/or 37.5 mg venlafaxine XR) (Table 22).

Antidepressant doses in GAD	
Paroxetine:	20–40 mg/day (occasionally 50–60 mg/day)
Venlafaxine:	75–150 mg/day (occasionally 225–300 mg/day)
Others:	Imipramine: 100–150 mg/day
	Other SSRIs: Routine doses

Table 21. Antidepressant doses in GAD.

Comparison of medications in GAD

	BZ	Buspirone	TCAs	SSRI/SNRI
Onset	Week 1	Week 2–4	Week 4–6	Week 2–4
Withdrawal symptoms	Yes	No	<10%	<10%
Abuse liability	Low/moderate	No	No	No
Alcohol interaction	Marked	Slight	Some	None
Sedation	Yes	No	Yes	No
Memory problems	Yes	No	Some	No
Cardiovascular effects	No	No	Yes	No
Cause depression	Occasionally	No	No	No
Treat/prevent depression	No	Perhaps	Yes	Yes
Dizziness	No	Yes	Yes	Occasionally
Insomnia	No	Sometimes	No	Yes
Nausea	No	Sometimes	No	Yes
Sexual side-effects	Yes	Sometimes	Yes	Commonly

Table 22. Comparison of medications in GAD (adapted with permission from reference 59).

Recommendations for pharmacotherapy

After the diagnosis of GAD and the need for pharmacotherapy is determined, current recommendations are that an SSRI, probably paroxetine, or an SNRI, probably venlafaxine, should be utilized in the long-term treatment of GAD.[31]

Length of treatment

If efficacy is observed and side-effects tolerable, the recommendation is that medications should be continued for at least six months to determine maximal effect (see below). To maintain efficacy and perhaps to prevent future depressive episodes, current recommendations are that treatment can be continued for 12–18 months before consideration of a slow taper and discontinuation. In the absence of studies to provide direct evidence, these recommendations are the result of a consensus among experts[31], largely based on the long-term safety of the use of antidepressants, increasing efficacy over time and probable prophylaxis against onset or recurrence of depression.

Long-term therapy

Two important long-term trials with paroxetine and venlafaxine XR have recently changed practice patterns in GAD. In two long-term follow-ups of patients initially treated for 8 weeks, but treatment continued for up to 6 months, the number of patients who ultimately had symptom remission continued to increase quite significantly at least up to month six. This meant that the number of patients who actually remitted and lost most or all of their symptoms rose from 25–40% in the short-term, to 65–70% over a 6-month trial. Therefore, if patients show even partial responses at a short-term 8-week trial, continued treatment at sufficient doses (20–40 mg paroxetine, 75–100 mg venlafaxine) should be continued for 6 months to determine ultimate response. It is these results, coupled with maintenance of response as long as treatment is continued and long-term prophylaxis against depression, that leads to the recommendations of routine treatment for 6–18 months with antidepressants (SSRI/SNRI) in GAD.

Psychological treatments

Cognitive behavioural therapy

Typically with CBT, patients are first asked to pay attention to the cues in their lives that they observe to trigger anxiety responses, as well as to their thoughts at the time. Patients are frequently taught relaxation techniques involving diaphragmatic breathing, muscle relaxation, meditation, etc. and are asked to practice these to reliably create a relaxation response. They are then asked to pair these relaxation responses to the cues and anxiety responses they find in their daily lives.

Another element in typical CBT involves the recognition and then challenge of the unrealistic and catastrophic thinking and worrying. These are challenged by helping the patient examine the objective accuracy or inaccuracy of these cognitions and subsequently generating cognitions that are in fact more accurate.[71]

Controlled trials

In a review of 35 controlled trials of various types of CBT,[72] Gould and colleagues reported overall greater efficacy than waiting list, anxiety management or nondirective therapies. A one-year follow-up found that CBT was associated with better outcomes than traditional analytic psychotherapy or other anxiety management type techniques.[73] In a review of 13 well-controlled, double-blind CBT trials, Borkovec demonstrated that CBT was superior to no treatment or nonspecific treatment and clearly demonstrated the effectiveness of CBT in GAD. The gains with short-term therapy with CBT were also maintained or actually increased over time.[71] These treatments are effective and in one trial even produced reductions in comorbid conditions at 12 months.[74]

Despite the clear demonstration of efficacy of CBT, therapists experienced in using CBT in GAD are uncommon even in psychiatric settings, and exceedingly rare in primary care. This makes it necessary for simpler psychotherapy techniques to be used in primary care, e.g. relaxation methods, supportive care and problem solving.[75] Although it is not yet demonstrated whether this particular therapy is effective in GA as depression, problem solving is certainly easier to teach to primary care clinicians and practice nurses, but again it is usually administered by specialist mental health professionals.

Combined pharmacological and psychological treatment

Unfortunately, it is unclear whether there is an advantage to combining medications and psychological treatments in patients with GAD.[76] In one study, concomitant treatment with BZ actually greatly reduced the efficacy of behaviour therapy and cognitive therapy (8% BZ, 86% without).[77] In contrast, a primary care 10-week study found that the combination of diazepam and CBT was more effective than either treatment alone.[78]

Obsessive Compulsive Disorder

Introduction

Although this puzzling and often debilitating disorder has been described for over a century, great progress has occurred in the last decade. This progress has primarily been driven by increased understanding that this is not a rare disorder but is surprisingly prevalent with a lifetime prevalence of 2–3%. Increased public and professional recognition has led to a marked increase in patients presenting for treatment. Although not commonly seen or treated in primary care, patients do present to their primary care physician with certain characteristic symptoms (see below).

Clinical picture

The clinical symptoms of OCD are primarily obsessions and compulsions. Obsessions are thoughts and images that repetitively intrude into the patient's thinking and are inappropriate and disturbing. Compulsions are the behaviours that are repeated many times in an attempt to reduce the anxiety related to obsessions (e.g. handwashing due to obsessive thoughts of being contaminated). The most prominent obsessions concern contamination, aggression, religiosity, symmetry, hoarding and sexual or religious thoughts. Compulsions include cleaning or washing, checking, arranging, hoarding and counting (Table 23).[79]

The most common obsession is certainly contamination, followed by obsessional pathological doubt (e.g. "did I turn off the iron or stove"), somatic obsessions and need for symmetry, e.g. with clothes, shoes, etc.

The most common compulsion is to check (e.g. stove, iron, front door lock, etc.), closely followed by washing and then counting and pressure to "confess". Many patients have compulsive rituals about how they eat their food, arrange clothes, etc. Others horde newspapers, rubbish, etc. Most patients have multiple obsessions that change over time.

Subtypes

Tic disorder

Probably the most important subtype is when OCD occurs with various tic disorders. These typically occur in more treatment resistant patients who frequently need the addition of neuroleptics to the SSRIs for effective treatment.[80]

Contamination fears

A common obsession is of contamination, usually of dirt, faeces or germs (e.g. AIDS). Patients may excessively wash, at times for many hours each day after they think they have touched a "contaminated object". Typically they also phobically avoid touching such items.

OCD symptoms on admission			
Obsessions	**%**	**Compulsions**	**%**
Contamination	50	Checking	61
Pathological doubt	42	Washing	50
Somatic	33	Counting	36
Need for symmetry	32	Need to ask or confess	34
Aggressive	31	Symmetry and precision	28
Sexual	24	Hoarding	18
Multiple obsessions	72	Multiple compulsions	58

Table 23. OCD symptoms on admission. Reprinted with permission from reference 79. Copyright 2002 American Psychiatric Association (www.appi.org)

Need for symmetry

Patients in this subtype feel driven to perform certain behaviours in a particular order or to arrange items in "a perfectly arranged" manner. This is often connected to magical thoughts that they may hurt loved ones if they fail to perform these actions correctly. Others may spend hours arranging items in their wardrobe or sock drawer until it feels "just right".

Some patients have what is thought to be a primary obsessional slowness and take an extremely long time to complete simple tasks (e.g. shaving, showering, etc.).

Pathological doubt

Patients worry that they have not done or forgotten to do something that will lead to a very negative outcome. These most commonly occur as a fear of not having turned off the stove or iron or locked the door. Often many patients may return home multiple times to check that they did it properly.

Somatic obsessions

Certainly the most common is a fear of having developed cancer or venereal disease, and, in the modern era, an irrational worry of having developed AIDS.

Sexual/aggressive

Patients may worry that they have run over someone when they hit a bump in the road. Some even confess that they may have committed a crime that they read about in the newspaper and others that they "might" do something like harm a child or stab someone with a kitchen knife.

Diagnosis

The diagnosis of OCD (as shown in Table 24) is based on recurrent obsessions (thoughts, impulses or images) that a person attempts to ignore, suppress or neutralize, which they realize are their own unwanted thoughts. The other diagnostic point is that these obsessions are paired with repetitive behaviours or mental acts that the person feels compelled to repeat in response to their obsessions in a rigid, ritualistic fashion. These behaviours are repeated to prevent some imagined bad outcome but are clearly recognized as excessive and time consuming (greater than one hour per day) and interfere significantly with the person's functioning.

Differential diagnosis

Since there are almost no disorders that produce similar symptoms to OCD, the differential diagnosis is generally not difficult except with comorbid tic disorders and the other frequently comorbid condition of depression (Table 25). Tic disorders commonly involve facial tics or involuntary sudden

DSM-IV-TR diagnostic criteria for OCD

A. Either obsessions or compulsions

Obsessions as defined by (1), (2), (3) and (4):

    (1) recurrent and persistent thoughts, impulses or images that are experienced, at some time during the disturbance, as intrusive and inappropriate and that cause marked anxiety or distress

    (2) the thoughts, impulses or images are not simply excessive worries about real-life problems

    (3) the person attempts to ignore or suppress such thoughts, impulses or images, or to neutralize them with some thought or action

    (4) the person recognizes that the obsessional thoughts, impulses, or images are a product of his or her own mind ____ imposed from without as in thought insertion

Compulsions as defined by (1) and (2):

    (1) repetitive behaviours (e.g. hand washing, ordering checking) or mental acts (e.g. praying, counting repeating silently) that the person feels driven to perform in response to an obsession, or according to rules that must be _____ rigidly

    (2) the behaviours or mental acts are aimed at preventing or reducing distress or preventing some dreaded event or situation; however, these behaviours or mental acts either are not connected in a realistic way with what they are designed to neutralize or prevent or are clearly excessive

Table 24. DSM-IV-TR diagnostic criteria for OCD. Reprinted with permission from the *Diagnostic and Statistical Manual of Mental Disorder, Fourth Edition*, Text Revision. Copyright 2000 American Psychatric Association (www.appi.org).

movements, generally grimaces or twitches. In its most complete form of Tourette's, tics are frequently combined with oral sounds, either grunts or fully formed words or phrases, which are frequently obscene. These involuntary movements are not accompanied by mental obsessions and are therefore not purposeful.

As most patients (two-thirds) with OCD also have a lifetime history of depression, and one-third are currently depressed, depression can be a complicating diagnostic feature. Most develop depression after OCD and, if

B. At some point during the course of the disorder, the person has recognized that the obsessions or compulsions are excessive or unreasonable. **Note:** This does not apply to children

C. The obsessions or compulsions cause marked distress, are time-consuming (take more than 1 hour a day), or significantly interfere with the person's normal routine, occupational (or academic) functioning, or usual social activities or relationships

D. If another axis 1 disorder is present, the content of the obsessions or compulsions is not restricted to it (e.g. preoccupation with food in the presence of an eating disorder; hair pulling in the presence of trichotillomania; concern with appearance in the presence of body dysmorphic disorder; preoccupation with drugs in the presence of a substance use disorder; _____ in the presence of a paraphilia; or guilty ruminations in the presence of a major depressive disorder)

E. The disturbance is not due to the direct physiological effects of a substance (e.g. a drug of abuse, a medication) or a general medical condition

Specify if:

With poor insight: if, for most of the time during the current episode, the person does not recognize that the obsessions and compulsions are excessive or unreasonable.

Differential diagnosis in OCD

Tic disorders (Tourette's)
Secondary depression
Schizophrenia with OCD symptoms
OCD comorbid with other anxiety disorders
Bipolar illness
Anorexia nervosa

Table 25. Differential diagnosis in OCD.

severe, can dominate the clinical picture. Generally, patients will be able to describe their development of OCD long before the development of depressive complications. OCD is frequently complicated by other anxiety disorders such as PD or social anxiety disorder, as well as bipolar disorder and eating disorders. Occasionally, individuals with schizophrenia will exhibit significant OCD symptoms and seem to have a particularly malignant form of psychosis and OCD.

Epidemiology

The National ECA Survey showed that the prevalence (6 months) of OCD was 1.6%, with a lifetime prevalence of 2.5%; thus, making OCD the fourth most common psychiatric disorder.[81] In the follow-up Cross-Cultural Study, lifetime rates of OCD across multiple cultures were remarkably consistent at 1.9–2.5% and annual rates 1.1–1.8% (Table 26).

It appears clear that there is a continuum of OCD symptoms, with a larger percentage having fewer symptoms and lower severity than those meeting the full clinical criteria. Interestingly, the subthreshold group is probably approximately 8%.[82]

Pathology

It is now clear that OCD is a heterogeneous disorder, with multiple subtypes based on different pathologies. These appear to involve genetic vulnerabilities, perhaps specific neuroanatomic abnormalities, immunology and potentially abnormalities of the serotonin system.

Genetics

Several studies have found that the concordance rates of OCD symptoms are over 80% for monozygotic pairs and approximately 50% for dizygotic twin pairs, thus suggesting a substantial genetic component. In recent family genetic studies, significantly higher rates of OCD symptoms were observed in first-degree relatives of probands with OCD for both full OCD (10.3% versus 1.9%) and subthreshold OCD (7.9% versus 2.0%), see Table 27.[83] There appear to be two groups of inherited risk for OCD: one at an early age in association with tic disorders and one that is not tic related.[83]

Epidemiology of OCD		
	Lifetime	**6-Month**
National ECA Survey	2.5%	1.6%
Cross-Cultural Study	1.9–2.5%	1.1–1.8% (annual)
*Note: subthreshold rates approximately 8%		

Table 26. Epidemiology of OCD.

Genetic findings in OCD	
Monozygotic concordance	80%+
Dizygotic concordance	50%
First-degree relatives with OCD symptoms	
Full OCD probands	10.3% (versus 1.9%)
Subthreshold OCD probands	7.9% (versus 2.0%)

Table 27. Genetic findings in OCD.

Neuroanatomical abnormalities

A series of elegant neuroimaging studies suggest that neuroanatomical abnormalities are involved with prefrontal cortical areas, striatum, thalamus and the reciprocal connections from the thalamus to the same prefrontal regions (Figure 3). Current models suggest that over activity in the orbitofrontal, prelimbic areas, which control response inhibition, flexibility and perseveration, is coupled with positive feedback loops between the cortex and thalamic circuits, which are thought to mediate circular repetitive thoughts. Abnormalities of this circuit may be responsible for the repetitive, ritualistic behaviours and compulsions. Although this hypothesis has considerable support from functional neuroimaging and neuropsychological testing, its only clinical usefulness at this point is that successful neurosurgical procedures appear to interrupt this circuit at the level of the internal capsule. This is also consistent with treatments that may inhibit cortical excitability, including the SSRIs, BZs and gabapentin (see below).

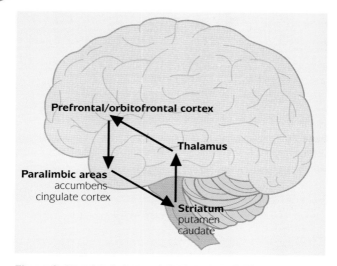

Figure 3. Postulated abnormal CNS circuit in OCD.

Serotonin

The primary evidence suggesting serotonin abnormalities in OCD is that SSRIs have such uniquely beneficial effects. Presumably, they work by down regulating 5-HT$_2$ autoregulators in the orbitofronto cortex. This would increase 5-HT activity and, therefore, inhibition in that region, which is postulated to be overactive in OCD.

Autoimmune disorders

Coupled with the observation that a minority of patients with Sydenham's chorea developed OCD and Tourette's symptoms, a certain number of children with an obsessional illness of abrupt onset and discrete episodes of symptom exacerbation appeared to have developed anti-neural antibodies to areas of the basal ganglia as part of an autoimmune response to an infection with group A-beta-haemolytic streptococcus. This has been called Paediatric Autoimmune Neuropsychiatric Disorder Associated with Streptococcal Infections or PANDAS[84] (Table 28). The possibility of early diagnosis and treatment, and even prophylaxis with antibiotics (and plasmaphoresis) makes early

Criteria for Paediatric Autoimmune Neuropsychiatric Disorders Associated with Streptococcal Infection (PANDAS)

(1) OCD and/or tic disorder
(2) Childhood/prepubertal onset
(3) Episodes of symptom increases
(4) Association with streptococcal infections
(5) Neurological abnormalities

Table 28. Criteria for Paediatric Autoimmune Neuropsychiatric Disorders Associated with Streptococcal Infection (PANDAS) (adapted from reference 84).

recognition of these children with sudden onset of OCD very important in primary care.

Physical examination

The physical examination of an OCD patient is generally normal unless the patient exhibits tics of comorbid Tourette's Disorder. However, patients may have physical findings related to their compulsive rituals, with the most common being red, chapped and chafed hands and arms from repeated washings. Evidence of other repetitive behaviours may be evident or the patient may be observed performing the rituals in the office (e.g. checking or counting rituals, arranging magazines in a particular order, or the need to ask or confess to something they fear they have done wrong).

Laboratory examinations

No expected abnormalities and, therefore, no tests suggested unless indicated from history or physical examination.

Age of onset

OCD usually begins in late adolescence or early 20s, but 21% of patients had onset before age 14 and 11% before age 12.[85]

Course

In general, the course of OCD is usually chronic with fluctuation in severity over time (Table 29). Recent studies suggest that (if followed prospectively) approximately 10–15% of patients will

Course of OCD	
Remission	10–15%
Episodic with partial remission	25%
Continuous but improving	25%
Continuous and unchanging	25%
Chronic deteriorating	14%

Table 29. Course of OCD.

enjoy a remission, while approximately 25% have an episodic course with partial remission, another 25% experience a continuous, unchanging course and a further 25% experience a continuous course but with improvement and a smaller group (14%) appears to have a chronic, deteriorating course without treatment.[86] With treatment (see below) some studies suggest that as many as 10–25% of patients recover or have only subclinical OCD symptoms (25%).

Pharmacotherapy

SSRIs

Certainly, the principal treatment for OCD is a trial of one of the SSRIs (with higher doses). However, the modern treatment of OCD began with the tricyclic derivative clomipramine, which appears to be uniquely effective among the tricyclics, probably because of its marked potential to block serotonin reuptake like the SSRIs. Although it remains one of the more effective pharmacotherapies for OCD, its greater side-effects (than SSRIs) have relegated it to a second-line treatment. It is clear that other antidepressants than clomipramine are not as effective as the SSRIs.

Four of the SSRIs (fluvoxamine, fluoxetine, paroxetine and sertraline) have FDA indications for OCD and citalopram has been shown to be efficacious in OCD. Efficacy in children has been demonstrated for fluvoxamine and sertraline and is assumed for the others.

Treatment

Initial treatment with an SSRI requires an adequate dose (often higher than the treatment for depression) for at least 10–12 weeks, because the therapeutic response of OCD is generally slower. The initial choice of an SSRI is dictated by expected side-effects and pharmacokinetic considerations because they all appear to be roughly equivalent in terms of efficacy. The dose can be increased every 3–7 days, limited only by initial side-effects, usually mild to moderate nausea. Occasionally, an SSRI can be either sedating or activating and should be given in the evening or morning depending upon patient feedback.

Suggested doses

Studies indicated optimal responses with paroxetine 40–60 mg, fluoxetine 40–60 mg, fluvoxamine 150 mg, sertraline 150 mg (Table 30). Higher doses are used by many experts if the response is only partial.

Perhaps the most critical issue in the initial phase of treatment is ensuring compliance with long-term treatment and the switches between SSRIs that may be required if the patient fails to response to the first, second or even third SSRI.

Long-term treatment

Patients are routinely treated for at least 1 year because if medication is discontinued relapse can be as high as 90%.[87]

Doses effective in OCD*	
Paroxetine	40–60 mg/d
Fluoxetine	40–60 mg/d
Fluvoxamine	150 mg/d
Sertraline	150 mg/d
Citalopram	40 mg
Clomipramine	150 (to 250 mg/d)
*Note: (1) Higher doses have been successful in treating some patients; (2) all can be given once daily except fluvoxamine (bid) and clomipramine (bid).	

Table 30. Doses effective in OCD.

However, evidence suggests that many patients can be successfully maintained on treatment at lower doses.[88]

Expected response

Although only approximately 10–15% of patients can expect a remission of symptoms, 70% of patients in most modern studies experience a clinically significant reduction in symptoms. This has frequently been described as a 25–35% decrease in scores on the Yale–Brown Obsessive Compulsive Scale (Y-BOCS).

Treatment strategy

If patients have a partial response, the recommendation is generally to attempt to find an augmenting treatment that will result in greater efficacy rather than switch to another SSRI. Recent data suggest that many patients continue to improve as treatment continues for 9–12 months (at least). However, if there has been no improvement, a trial with a second SSRI would be recommended.

Positive responses with augmentation have been reported with tryptophan, fenfluramine, lithium, buspirone, clonazepam, pindolol or adding a second SSRI or SNRI, such as venlafaxine. Other approaches have suggested adding an antipsychotic medication, either a traditional one like haloperidol or preferably a newer atypical antipsychotic, such as risperidone. All of these strategies are associated with significant side-effects and the necessity to use them should probably lead to a specialty referral.

Specialist referral

As mentioned above, the use of complicated pharmacotherapeutic regimens, either in terms of very high doses or combination treatment, is a primary reason for specialist referral (Table 31). Failure to respond to either one or two SSRIs suggests a treatment refractory OCD illness. The therapeutic manoeuvres to treat these patients include high doses and combination therapy, as well as other treatments that have shown promise, including intravenous clomipramine, rapid transcranial magnetic stimulation and neurosurgery. There have been multiple studies of successful neurosurgical treatment of intractable and treatment-resistant OCD, generally including internal capsule lesions. This currently

Reasons for specialist referral of OCD patient

A. Poor response to initial treatment (one or two SSRIs)

B. Need for:
   (1) High dose pharmacotherapy
   (2) Combination pharmacotherapy
   (3) IV clomipramine
   (4) Behaviour therapy (response/prevention)
   (5) Rapid transcranial magnetic stimulation (rTMS)
   (6) Neurosurgery

C. Comorbidity (Tourette's or tic disorder, schizophrenia, bipolar disorder, anorexia nervosa, complex PD, or social anxiety disorder)

Table 31. Reasons for specialist referral of OCD patient.

includes the bloodless gamma knife techniques, and all of these techniques should be considered before considering a patient treatment resistant.

Summary

The frequently complex behavioural treatments of OCD are another common reason for specialist referral. Recommended treatment is with an SSRI, with an initial treatment period of 12–16 weeks and doses higher than those utilized for the treatment of depression. Most patients are treated for 1–2 years before consideration of a slow taper and discontinuation. Because relapse is quite high, many patients are treated indefinitely, particularly if they have experienced a positive response and few side-effects and/or previous relapses.

Psychotherapy

Somewhat surprisingly, controlled trials of behaviour therapy suggest that it is at least as effective as pharmacotherapy and probably more effective even in short-term treatment. For instance when a 50% improvement is required on the Y–BOCS (higher than many pharmacotherapy trials) fully 75% of patients appear to respond. Improvements are routinely either maintained or extended in long-term follow-up and are maintained and not lost when patients discontinue formal behaviour therapy.

Description of behaviour therapy

Patients are initially helped to recognize what triggers their obsessions and compulsions and then asked to arrange them in increasing severity prior to systematic exposure to these triggers. They then need to be educated on the therapeutic rationale of exposure in vivo but with prevention of their usual ritual/response, which leads to habituation. In collaboration with the therapist, patients agree to begin exposure and ritual prevention. Sessions typically range from 15 minutes to as much as a few hours.

Exposure and response (ritual) prevention can occur gradually with spaced practice, or in intensive programmes requiring many hours per day and multiple days per week. Now, there are also evolving programmes for self-help exposure and response prevention treatments, either occurring with the help of a manual or computer programs. Perhaps the best developed programme has been by Marks and colleagues[89] and is called BT-STEPS. This is an interactive system using a telephone and a workbook that allows the design and implementation of a self-help programme and has been demonstrated to be effective.

Behaviour therapy and pharmacotherapy

At least one-quarter of patients routinely refuse behaviour therapy, fearing that it will be too anxiety provoking. Many of these patients are willing to take medication. In this case, initial treatment with an SSRI can lead to a preparation of the patient for effective behaviour therapy and their effects appear to be additive.

Specialist referral

Behaviour therapists skilled in the techniques for treating OCD are not widely available. Referral for behaviour therapy should generally be considered in any patient who prefers nonpharmacological treatment. If the patient is initially treated unsuccessfully with pharmacotherapy in the primary care setting, a specialist referral should be considered for behaviour therapy or complex psychopharmacology.

Social Anxiety Disorder (Social Phobia)

Introduction

Although social anxiety disorder or social phobia may well be the most prevalent anxiety disorder (lifetime 13%), it is certainly the least well understood and recognized. Several surveys suggest that approximately 7% of primary care patients have this disorder, but in both those studies in San Diego and Paris,[90,91] none of the patients were recognized to have this disorder by their primary care physician.

Social anxiety disorder is also misunderstood to be only a minor disorder or is mistaken for shyness. As described below, it is quite a severe disorder, and can literally dominate and destroy the lives of people who develop it, frequently in childhood. Although there is some waxing and waning, generally social anxiety of this severity continues to worsen over time unless treated.

Clinical picture

Individuals with this disorder have excessive anxiety and fear in social situations, fearing that observers will think badly of them because they observe them to be nervous, anxious, blushing, hand-shaking, etc. These anxieties can occur in many social situations, including parties, shopping, talking with strangers, such as a salesperson in a shop, talking to the boss at work or giving presentations in a work or social setting (Table 32). Because this anxiety is so severe, individuals avoid these situations or endure them with a great deal of distress. They might also have a severe PA if forced into these situations.

Subtypes

The most important grouping is the generalized subtype for people who fear and avoid many social situations or fear

Subtypes of social anxiety disorder (social phobia)

Generalized
To "most" social situations:
    Parties
    Eating in public
    Talking to sales assistants
    Approaching a group of strangers
    Dating or asking for a date
    Talking to employer
    Job requiring interaction with strangers
    Classroom interactions
Circumscribed (specific)
To one (or two) situations only:
    Public speaking
    Signing one's name in front of others
    Using public toilet

Table 32. Subtypes of social anxiety disorder (social phobia).

situations where they might have to perform or where they have to interact (e.g. at a party, asking directions of strangers). This subtype is associated with the greatest severity, dysfunction and generally earliest onset. A statistically larger group are those who only have one or perhaps two feared situations and they are generally described as having limited (specific, discrete or circumscribed) social phobias. One of the most common is giving a speech, but this subtype also involves individuals with isolated difficulties like eating in public, using a public lavatory, writing a cheque in public (see Table 32).

Diagnosis

Diagnostic criteria for social phobia (social anxiety disorder) are listed in Table 33 and involve the "marked and persistent fear" of social situations where a person will be scrutinized by others and fears that it will be "humiliating or embarrassing". Exposure to these feared situations can lead to PAs, and these situations are either avoided altogether, endured with distress or the patient consumes alcohol to reduce this anxiety prior to the social situation. Patients recognize these fears as excessive and unreasonable, although they may mistakenly conclude that it is "just part of my personality".

Differential diagnosis

This disorder most closely resembles PD, in which similar anxiety can occur and often does occur in crowds, perhaps even around public speaking. The primary differentiating point is that the anxiety in social anxiety is always in social situations, whereas in PD the PAs can occur when the patient is alone or even at home or in the supermarket when there is little or no social interaction. Also, the thoughts of the PD patient are about having another horrible PA, whereas the social anxiety patient thinks principally that they will be humiliated or embarrassed in front of another person, and that is their fear.

Individuals with PTSD often fear interactions with other people, but only in relationship to the previous trauma. The GAD patient may have concerns about interactions with others, but generally this has to do with their worries about everything or that they will need to be "perfect" in front of others.

Certainly the withdrawal of many individuals with this disorder can be confused with the isolation of PD patients (agoraphobia), but again this is related to a fear of PAs occurring when an individual leaves the home. Isolation seen in very depressed patients can be differentiated because of the other signs of severe depression, e.g. crying, sleep disturbances, weight changes, etc.

Epidemiology

Although earliest studies suggested a prevalence rate perhaps as low as 2.4%, more recent studies have suggested that the lifetime prevalence rate is actually 13%, making only depression and alcohol dependence more common.[5] These rates appear to be similar across ethnic groups and in most developed nations, certainly including the US, Canada and Europe.

DSM-IV diagnostic criteria for social phobia

A. A marked and persistent fear of one or more social or performance situations in which the person is exposed to unfamiliar people or to possible scrutiny by others. The individual fears that he or she will act in a way (or show anxiety symptoms) that will be humiliating or embarrassing. **Note:** In children, there must be evidence of the capacity for age-appropriate social relationships with familiar people and the anxiety must occur in peer settings, not just in interactions with adults

B. Exposure to the feared social situation almost invariably provokes anxiety, which may take the form of a situationally bound or situationally predisposed PA. Note: In children, the anxiety may be expressed by crying, tantrums, freezing, or shrinking from social situations with unfamiliar people

C. The person recognizes that the fear is excessive or unreasonable. **Note:** In children, this feature may be absent

D. The feared social or performance situations are avoided or else are endured with intense anxiety or distress

E. The avoidance, anxious anticipation, or distress in the feared social or performance situation(s) interferes significantly with the person's normal routine, occupational (academic) functioning, or social activities or relationships, or there is marked distress about having the phobia

F. In individuals under age 18 years, the duration is at least 6 months

G. The fear or avoidance is not due to the direct physiological effects of a substance (e.g. a drug of abuse, a medication) or a general medical condition and is not better accounted for by another mental disorder (e.g. PD with or without agoraphobia, separation anxiety disorder, body dysmorphic disorder, a pervasive developmental disorder, or schizoid personality disorder)

H. If a general medical condition or another mental disorder is present, the fear in Criterion A is unrelated to it, e.g. the fear is not of stuttering, trembling in Parkinson's disease, or exhibiting abnormal eating behaviour in anorexia nervosa or bulimia nervosa

Specify if:

Generalized: if the fears include most social situations (also consider the additional diagnosis of avoidant personality disorder)

Table 33. DSM-IV diagnostic criteria for social phobia. Reprinted with permission from the *Diagnostic and Statistical Manual of Mental Disorder, Fourth Edition*, Text Revision. Copyright 2000 American Psychatric Association (www.appi.org).

Comorbidity

Most (80–90%) patients with social anxiety disorder have one or more comorbid conditions, either major depression, another anxiety disorder or a substance abuse disorder. Epidemiology in primary care settings suggests that 5–10% of patients suffer from this disorder. As mentioned, specific studies[90,91] indicate that 7% of patients in the primary care/general medicine setting met rigid diagnostic criteria for social anxiety disorder. Unfortunately, in these studies in San Diego and Paris, none of these patients were recognized to have this disorder by their clinician, underscoring the need for increased recognition and treatment of this disorder.

Pathology

Higher rates of social phobia are found in the relatives of individuals with social phobia (16% versus 5%).[92] An even higher rate was found in a recent study (26.4% versus 12.7%) when probands with generalized social phobia were studied.[93] Twin studies suggest that 30-40% of the risk for social phobia is genetic,[94] but no linkage studies have been completed (Table 34).

Neurobiology

Again, studies have suggested NE and particularly serotonin abnormalities in social anxiety. Interestingly, dopamine abnormalities have also been implicated, coupled with decreases

Genetic evidence in social anxiety disorder	
Family studies	
Higher rates in first-degree relatives	16% versus 5%
Even higher in relatives of generalized subtype	26.4% versus 2.7%
Twin studies suggest heritability	30–40%

Table 34. Genetic evidence in social anxiety disorder.

in putamen volume. Tihonen and colleagues reported (using SPECT) that patients with this disorder had markedly lower dopamine reuptake sites in the striatum.[95] It has been found that patients with a social anxiety challenge paradigm had an increased blood flow to the left superior anterior cingulate and medial frontal cortex areas and decreased flow to temporal pole, pons and left amygdala.

Physical examination/laboratory examination

No abnormalities are expected or have been found.

Pharmacotherapy

SSRIs

Certainly SSRIs are the treatment of choice for pharmacological treatment of social anxiety disorder. Large international, multi-centre, double-blind, placebo-controlled trials have been completed with paroxetine in which 55% of patients were classified as responders versus 24% on placebo. Decreases on the Liebowitz Social Anxiety Scale (LSAS) in these trials generally fell from the very severe range to the mild moderate range, and patients in the moderate level at baseline generally fell to the mildly symptomatic range.[96] A subsequent large trial by Baldwin found a similar response (66% versus 32%).[70]

In similar trials, fluvoxamine was shown to be effective with 47% versus 7% responding in one trial[90] and van Vliet and colleagues found 43% versus 23%.[97] Although there are no placebo-controlled trials published with fluoxetine, open small trials suggest that it is effective.

Dose

Doses of fluoxetine have been up to 50 mg with no clear dose determined but is generally used in range 20–60 mg/day (see Table 35). Sertraline was utilized up to 200 mg/day (mean dose of 123.5 mg/day) in one open trial. In an open trial of paroxetine the mean dose was 47.9 mg/day. Fluvoxamine is frequently used in the range 100–250 mg, and in one open trial[90] the mean dose was 202 mg/day.

SSRI doses in social anxiety disorder (social phobia)	
Paroxetine	20–50 mg/d
Sertraline	50–200 mg/d
Fluvoxamine	100–250 mg/d
Fluoxetine	20–60 mg/d

Table 35. SSRI doses in social anxiety disorder (social phobia).

BZs

The best-studied BZ has certainly been clonazepam, with several open trials and one large placebo-controlled trial. In this trial[98] 78% of patients responded, compared with 20% on placebo.

In an open trial, alprazolam showed some promise, but in the only double-blind study[99] it was less effective than the MAOI phenelzine.

Clonazepam has been generally utilized in the 0.5–3 mg/day range, averaging 2.0–4.3 mg/day. Alprazolam has been studied in the range of 1–8 mg/day.

Traditional (irreversible) MAOIs

One of the best-studied MAOIs is phenelzine with several double-blind, placebo-controlled trials demonstrating its efficacy. Its response rates were 64% versus 23%[100] and 69% versus 20% in the trial mentioned above.[99] In subsequent trials response rates as high as 91% were observed. Mean doses in these trials were 75.7, 55 and 67.5 mg/day. Open studies with tranylcypromine also suggest that it is effective.

Reversible MAOIs

Studies with reversible MAOIs are promising because special low tyramine diets are not required and side-effects are considerably lower than the traditional MAOI. Brofaromine has been shown in placebo-controlled trials to be effective (80% versus 14% and 78% versus 23%)[101] with large decreases in LSAS scores. In a recent trial,[102] brofaromine utilized at a mean dose of 107.2 mg/day in divided doses had 50% versus 19%

of patients rated as "much or very much improved" at endpoint. There have been four double-blind trials with moclobemide, one showing strong efficacy, one showing weak efficacy and two showing no clinically significant effects. In one trial,[103] moclobemide appeared to be as effective as phenelzine except on avoidance; however, subsequent published and unpublished trials would suggest that moclobemide is associated with modest efficacy at best. Unfortunately only meclobemide is available and only in certain countries.

Beta-adrenergic blockers
Although widely utilized by performers (e.g. violinists) who report positive results, beta-blockers in clinical trials with patients with generalized social anxiety fail to show any significant efficacy. In the controlled trial mentioned above[100] comparing placebo to phenelzine and atenolol (97.6 mg/day), the beta-blocker failed to show efficacy. In a subsequent controlled trial[104] significant efficacy for atenolol again was not demonstrated. In fact, a recent consensus group suggested that despite their popularity in general medicine, beta-blockers should not be utilized in social anxiety,[105] except in performers with no anxiety symptoms.

Other medications
Buspirone has been demonstrated to be effective in smaller open trials with response rates in the 45–70% range. Interestingly, controlled trials of buspirone have failed to show efficacy. The promising open trials did utilize higher doses, suggesting that perhaps 60 mg/day might be effective. The limited evidence with TCAs is that they are ineffective, including clomipramine.

Medication choice
Non-generalized social phobia arising only in specific and infrequent situations (e.g. musicians, professional talks) can be successfully treated with beta-blockers used only as a prn basis. A BZ like clonazepam could also be utilized in similar "prn" situations.

However, generalized social anxiety is generally long-term and chronic so the SSRIs are generally recommended. In countries where brofaromine is available, it is certainly a good first or second option. Most would not recommend the use of irreversible MAOIs unless other treatments have failed and this is a good indication for specialist referral. Clonazepam may be utilized as a second option as well.[105]

Psychotherapy

Exposure treatments

Repeated exposure to feared social situations has been long known to be an essential ingredient for effective psychotherapies of this disorder. There is some question that exposure alone is sufficient[106] and, more typically, exposure techniques have been combined with cognitive techniques or with social effectiveness training. In small studies, social effectiveness training has been shown to be effective in over 80% of patients.[107]

Exposure treatments and CBT

Techniques combining exposure and cognitive restructuring have been widely studied and shown to be effective. Probably the most studied technique has been developed for treatment of social phobia in a group setting using CBT (CBGT).[108] Combination therapy with phenelzine (MAOI) utilizing this CBGT was recently studied in a large randomized trial comparing phenelzine with CBGT and placebo for 12 weeks. The results showed that 75% of CBGT patients, 77% of phenelzine patients and 31% of placebo patients were rated as responders. Medication responders had greater improvement than CBGT responders, although following discontinuation of the medication, there were greater maintenance of gains from the CBGT group than the phenelzine group. Whether combination medication and CGBT would be more efficacious than either treatment alone is currently under study.

Other psychosocial treatments

Ongoing trials suggest that interpersonal psychotherapy, which has been shown to be effective in depression, also leads to positive results in social anxiety disorder,[109] with as many as 78% responding in one trial.

Summary

CBT techniques involve exposure to feared situations. They are perhaps best used in group settings where social activities can be practised and have been shown to be highly effective. Unfortunately, these specific treatments are not widely available and almost always require referral for specialist treatment.

Overall treatment recommendations

For most patients with a single social phobia for public speaking or anxiety during a single performance situation, prn beta-blockers or clonazepam might be effective. However, most patients with generalized social anxiety have had this disorder for generally 10–20 years with serious disruption of their lives. In that context, the recommendation is to use an SSRI with or without clonazepam. In patients who do not have adequate response to an SSRI alone, clonazepam or buspirone addition might be considered, followed by a trial with an MAOI, either the reversible MAOI brofaromine if available, or phenelzine.

Outpatients should be encouraged to gradually re-expose themselves to situations in which they are fearful and are avoiding. Formal psychotherapy, principally CBT, is effective and when available or preferred by the patient, should be utilized. It is still unclear if the combination of these two approaches is preferable.

If medications are to be utilized, current recommendations are to utilize them for 1–2 years if effective before considering a slow taper and discontinuation. Social fears inhibiting children from speaking up in classroom has been shown to lead to foreshortened educational careers. Also social development is retarded, particularly in forming relationships with the opposite sex, often resulting in lower rates of marriage. These same fears interfere with work situations. Occupational success is also reduced. For these reasons, treatment of children with this disorder is recommended although this remains a controversial topic.

Post-Traumatic Stress Disorder

Introduction

Emotional reactions to trauma were first explored through military trauma, although recently the importance of trauma in everyday civilian life has become increasingly recognized both because of their high frequency and of the reaction we now call PTSD. We now know that over 60% of US citizens experience a trauma capable of producing PTSD. However, treatments are just beginning to be developed to deal with this level of trauma in our society and in our medical practices.

Clinical picture

The clinical features of PTSD occur in three main areas (Table 36):

- Re-experiencing of the trauma in flashbacks, nightmares, or intrusive memories.
- Avoidance of stimuli that remind one of the trauma, general numbing of responsiveness, attachment to

---

Main symptom areas in PTSD

Re-experiencing the trauma
    Nightmares
    Flashbacks
    Intrusive memories
Avoidance of reminders, stimuli and emotional feelings
    Avoidance of reminders (avoiding revisiting area of trauma, memories or thoughts about trauma, etc.)
    Emotional numbing or detachment
    Restriction of feelings of affection or pleasure
Increased arousal
    Exaggerated startle response
    Irritability
    Difficult sleep
    Poor concentration/memory

Table 36. Main symptom areas in PTSD.

others or the inability to remember important aspects of the event.

- Increased arousal, including exaggerated startle responses, poor sleep, difficulty concentrating, hypervigilance and irritability.

These symptoms occur after many types of trauma from rape to motor vehicle accidents to reactions to war-time trauma, and appear to represent a basic response to overwhelming trauma. Individuals are essentially trapped by their intense memories of the trauma and their feelings of helplessness and horror. This interferes with their daily lives to a remarkable degree. They try to forget but it is too traumatic. Forgetting is interrupted by involuntary re-experiencing of the memories. Patients attempt to numb themselves, interfering with their ongoing relationships. Over time the symptoms of hyperarousal are perhaps the most problematic. They interfere with the individual's need to "make sense" of what has happened to them because each reminder is so physiologically distressing.

There has been considerable controversy about which events are sufficient to cause PTSD. For years, the definition has been "a stressor that would be markedly distressing to almost anyone" and/or which is "outside the range of usual human experience". These have included not only war-time experiences but also natural disasters and deliberate man-made disasters like terrorism. They have also involved interpersonal violence, like rape or torture, but can also involve witnessing others' trauma, particularly relatives, and most frequently follow

Traumatic events leading to PTSD
Combat
Rape
Threat with a weapon
Physical attack involving serious injury or threat to physical integrity or death
Witnessing a traumatic event to friend, family, or loved one
Fire, flood
Motor vehicle accident

Table 37. Traumatic events leading to PTSD.

motor vehicle accidents. Almost always the event involves a "serious threat to one's life or physical integrity" or to others, family or friends (Table 37).

Recent diagnostic criteria in the DSM-IV (see Table 38) have added further clarification by stating that the individual "experienced, witnessed and/or was confronted by an event that involved actual or threatened death or serious injury". In

DSM-IV diagnostic criteria for post-traumatic

A. The person has been exposed to a traumatic event in which both of the following were present:

(1) the person experienced, witnessed or was confronted with an event or events that involved actual or threatened death or serious injury, or a threat to the physical integrity of self or others

(2) the person's response involved intense fear, helplessness, or horror. **Note:** In children, this may be expressed instead by disorganized or agitated behaviour

B. The traumatic event is persistently re-experienced in one (or more) of the following ways:

(1) recurrent and intrusive distressing recollections of the event, including images, thoughts, or perceptions. **Note:** In young children, repetitive play may occur in which themes or aspects of the trauma are exposed

(2) recurrent distressing dreams of the event. Note: In children, there may be frightening dreams without recognizable content

(3) acting or feeling as if the traumatic event were recurring (includes a sense of reliving the experience, illusions, hallucinations and dissociative flashback episodes, including those that occur on awakening or when intoxicated). **Note:** In young children, trauma-specific re-enactment may occur

(4) intense psychological distress at exposure to internal or external cues that symbolize or resemble an aspect of the traumatic event

(5) physiological reactivity on exposure to internal or external cues that symbolize or resemble an aspect of the traumatic event

C. Persistent avoidance of stimuli associated with the trauma and numbing of general responsiveness (not present before the trauma), as indicated by three (or more) of the following:

Table 38. DSM-IV diagnostic criteria for PTSD. Reprinted with permission from the *Diagnostic and Statistical Manual of Mental*

addition, it was added that the response "involved intense fear, helplessness, or horror," capturing that the critical aspect is the overwhelming reaction of the person.

Diagnosis

The diagnostic criteria require the so-called "A Criterion" of the trauma as described above. In addition, diagnosis requires that

stress disorder

(1) efforts to avoid thoughts, feelings or conversations associated with the trauma

(2) efforts to avoid activities, places or people that arouse recollections of the trauma

(3) inability to recall an important aspect of the trauma

(4) markedly diminished interest or participation in significant activities

(5) feeling of detachment or estrangement from others

(6) restricted range of affect (e.g. unable to have loving feelings)

(7) sense of a foreshortened future (e.g. does not expect to have a career, marriage, children, or a normal lifespan)

D. Persistent symptoms of increased arousal (not present before the trauma), as indicated by two (or more) of the following:

(1) difficulty falling or staying asleep

(2) irritability or outbursts of anger

(3) difficulty concentrating

(4) hypervigilance

(5) exaggerated startle response

E. Duration of the disturbance (symptoms in criteria B, C and D) is more than 1 month

F. The disturbance causes clinically significant distress or impairment in social, occupational, or other important areas of functioning

Specify if:

Acute: if duration of symptoms is less than 3 months

Chronic: if duration of symptoms is 3 months or more

Specify if:

With delayed onset: if onset of symptoms is at least 6 months after the stressor

the person re-experience the trauma in one or more ways (dreams, intrusive recollections, flashbacks, etc.), persistently avoid stimuli associated with the trauma indicated by three or more symptoms, such as avoiding thoughts, activities, reminders of the trauma or detachment from others or restricted range of affect (see Tables 36 and 37). The third criterion of increased arousal must be demonstrated by two or more symptoms, e.g. difficulty sleeping, irritability, concentration, startle reactions, etc. By definition, it has occurred for longer than 1 month and is clinically significant.

Differential diagnosis:

Although PTSD patients experience anxiety and PAs similar to other anxiety disorders, they also exhibit other characteristic symptoms (flashbacks, increased arousal) and the symptomatology begins after severe trauma.

Epidemiology

Although early studies suggested that the lifetime rate was 1.5%, more recent studies suggest a much higher rate. In a large HMO in Detroit, 39.1% of the sample was traumatized and the rate of those traumatized who developed PTSD was 23.6%. This resulted in an overall lifetime prevalence rate of 9.2%.[110] In other studies (see Table 39) 51% of women and 61% of men had been exposed to traumatic events, with 5% of men and 10.4% of women developing PTSD from these trauma (Table 40).[111] In active combat situations, 40–70% of men have been observed to develop some level of acute or chronic anxiety

Prevalence of traumatic events		
Trauma	**Male**	**Female**
Rape	0.7	9.2
Molestation	2.8	12.3
Physical attack	11.1	6.9
Combat	6.4	0.0
Accident	25.0	13.8
Disaster	18.9	15.2
Any trauma	60.7	51.2

Table 39. Prevalence of traumatic events.

and/or PTSD reaction. The best evaluation of veterans was the National Vietnam Veterans Readjustment Study.[112] In that sample, 15% of male veterans met full criteria for PTSD and an additional 11% had partial PTSD. Almost all studies show associations between the severity and duration of the combat exposure and PTSD. Certainly being wounded or involved in very traumatic experiences, such as mutilations and burial details, were associated with the highest rates. Rates in prisoners of war are 50–70% and victims of terrorist attacks are 20–40%. Studies of resettled refugees find PTSD rates that are close to 50%. Approximately 70% of victims of various types of violence, such as rape, homicides, sniper attacks and battered women, develop PTSD.

Probability of association between trauma experience and PTSD		
Trauma	**Male**	**Female**
Rape	65.0	45.9
Molestation	12.2	26.5
Physical attack	1.8	21.3
Combat	38.8	
Accident	22.3	48.5
Disaster	3.7	5.4
Any trauma	8.1	20.4
% PTSD	5.0	10.4

Table 40. Probability of association between trauma experience and PTSD.

Risk factors for PTSD

Severity of trauma
    - repeated/prolonged
    - fear of dying/serious injury
    - overwhelming vulnerability or loss of control
Childhood abuse/trauma
Pre-existing psychiatric illness
Family history of PTSD
Substance abuse
Low educational, socioeconomic status or social support

Table 41. Risk factors for PTSD.

Risk factors

The severity of the trauma appears to be the greatest risk factor for a person to develop PTSD followed by prior trauma, family history of PTSD and pre-existing psychiatric problems (Table 41).

Other psychiatric responses to trauma other than PTSD

As illustrated in Figure 4, the most common reaction to trauma is to develop no disorder. Although PTSD occurs in approximately one-third of trauma individuals who do develop a pathological reaction, almost equally common are other anxiety problems or depression.

Physiology

A series of studies have suggested that a complex disorder of the hypothalamic pituitary axis (HPA) that may be hypersensitive to stress in PTSD, with decreased cortisol release and an increased negative feedback inhibition.[113] This has been demonstrated by hypersecretion of CRF, blunting of the ACTH response to CRF and lower 24-hour urinary cortisol excretion, as well as increased lymphocyte and glucocorticoid receptors. Women visiting the emergency room hours after rape had lower cortisol levels if they had experienced a previous rape.[114] Similarly, it was found that recent motor vehicle accident victims with low cortisol levels were more likely to develop PTSD later.[115]

Catecholamine alteration

Studies are mixed, but some studies found increased NE measures after trauma and in PTSD. It was found that a patient's heart rate in the emergency room after a motor vehicle accident was higher in those who eventually developed PTSD at the 4-month follow-up.[116]

Overall biological model

It would appear that the acute HPA and sympathetic (NE) increases with stress become abnormal over time in the PTSD situation. It is postulated that the basic pathophysiologic

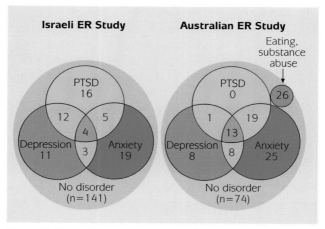

Figure 4. Psychiatric responses within 4–6 months post-trauma.

abnormality involves a failure to turn off the HPA axis and sympathetic system after stress.[117]

Physical examination

In addition to physical findings from the trauma itself, PTSD patients characteristically display increased startle reactions and increased pulse rates on physical examination.

Laboratory examination

No abnormalities are expected except potential changes in the cortisol system.

Clinical course

In those who do develop PTSD after trauma, approximately 50% lose their symptoms over the first 6 months (Figure 5). Nightmares typically move from explicit re-enactments of the trauma to less and less accurate repetitions of the trauma, to those accompanied by a sense of helplessness. Hopefully, flashbacks also wane with time. Perhaps the most persistent symptoms are the hyperarousal ones of increased startle reaction, difficulty sleeping and irritability.

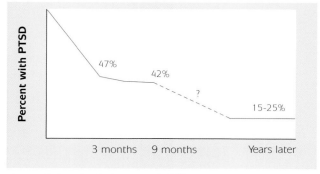

Figure 5. Longitudinal course of PTSD.

Common physical symptoms after trauma			
Course of Symptoms Following Rape (%)			
Symptom	**2 Weeks**	**1 Month**	**4 Months**	**1 Year**
Headaches	54	39	29	27
Nausea	44	38	20	22
Back pain	37	26	30	30
Allergies	31	13	22	16
Cardiac	30	23	18	20
Menstrual	27	21	20	16

Table 42. Common physical symptoms after trauma.

As outlined in Table 42, physical problems may very well persist, including headaches, nausea, back pain, etc. Unfortunately, PTSD becomes a chronic disorder in up to one-third of patients in some samples (Figure 5).

Pharmacotherapy (Table 43)
SSRIs
SSRIs have now been studied in multiple well-controlled trials over the last several years (Table 44).

In several trials with fluoxetine, PTSD symptoms were reduced, particularly arousal and numbing, as well as avoidance symptoms. As has been observed with other medications, combat-related PTSD appeared to be more treatment refractory.

Treatment goals in PTSD
Reduce PTSD symptoms Improve resilience to stress Improve quality of life Reduce disability Treat comorbidities

Table 43. Treatment goals in PTSD.

SSRI doses in PTSD	
SSRIs	
Fluoxetine	20–80 mg/d
Sertraline	50–200 mg/d
Paroxetine	20–50 mg/d (mean 42.5 mg/d)
Fluvoxamine	50–200 mg/d
Serotonin antagonist reuptake inhibitors	
Nefazodone	400–600 mg/d

Table 44. SSRI doses in PTSD.

Sertraline

A large 12-week double-blind trial of sertraline led to the first FDA approval in the US of a treatment for PTSD. Symptoms that improved included most of the PTSD symptoms, such as re-experiencing, hyperarousal, aggression and depression. Veterans did not respond as well to sertraline treatment. Paroxetine has recently been studied in large double-blind trials as well with seemingly broader response across all the symptom clusters (including combat trauma) and both men and women.[118]

Fluvoxamine has been studied in small trials and demonstrated to be effective in doses of 50–200 mg/day, with effectiveness across all PTSD clusters.

Serotonin antagonist reuptake inhibitors

Nefazodone has been shown to be effective across all the PTSD symptoms for veterans and civilian trauma victims, perhaps especially in the avoidance cluster[119] (Table 45).

Doses of other effective medications in PTSD

Tricyclics		
Amitriptyline	50–300 mg/d	
Imipramine	100–200 mg/d	
MAOIs		
Phenelzine	30–90 mg/d	
Buspirone	5–30 mg/d	
Anticonvulsants		
Carbamazepine	200–1000 mg/d (levels 8.4–11.5 mg/ml)	
Valproic acid	250–2000 mg/d (levels 44–103 mg/ml)	
Atypical antipsychotics		
Risperidone	5–10 mg/d	

Table 45. Doses of other effective medications in PTSD.

Tricyclic antidepressants

Desipramine, imipramine and amitriptyline have all been shown to be effective and, unlike some of the SSRIs, they have been particularly effective in veteran populations. Amitryptiline reduced not only PTSD symptoms but also depression and anxiety in veterans.[120]

Desipramine was relatively ineffective, showing efficacy only after the fourth week, probably because of the low dosages, whereas imipramine produced improvement in 65% of veterans (versus 28% placebo).

MAOIs

Phenelzine has been studied in several studies in combat veterans. In one study there was significantly greater improvement with phenelzine than imipramine or placebo, especially against intrusive symptoms.

Buspirone

Because buspirone does not share the abuse liability of the BZs, it was disappointing that trials to date have shown a poor response in this condition.

Mood stabilizers

These have been utilized based on the hypothesis that a kindling-like process may be involved in PTSD. Lithium has shown positive effects, particularly against rage, hyperarousal, numbing and over-reactivity to stress. Open trials of carbamazepine have shown benefit against intrusive symptoms, nightmares and flashbacks with promising results against other PTSD symptoms. A few studies suggest improvement with valproate. One small trial suggests improvement with lamotrigine against the symptoms of re-experiencing and avoidance/numbing.

Atypical antipsychotics

Pilot trials of both quetiapine and risperidone are promising. One controlled trial with risperidone was positive and one with olanzapine was negative.

Summary

The SSRIs would appear to be the treatment of choice in PTSD. If they are ineffective, the MAOI phenelzine (or brofaromine if available) is probably indicated. In some treatment-resistant patients, mood-stabilizing agents or anticonvulsants may be effective, as might atypical antipsychotics. In combat veterans, amitriptyline, imipramine and phenelzine have been shown to be particularly effective, although modern trials with paroxetine and other SSRIs suggest they are perhaps equally effective.

Psychotherapy

Although relatively well-developed, psychotherapies for PTSD are almost always beyond the primary care setting and an indication for specialist referral.

Rationale for psychotherapy

Patients are overwhelmed by the memories of the trauma and physiologic reactions to memories and unable to focus on their traumatic past. They need to regain control of their own emotional and physical responses and place the traumatic event in some larger perspective that allows them to realize that however traumatic it was, it should not recur. Patients also need:

- To develop a sense of safety in which they can think about the memories related to the trauma.
- To disconnect the extreme fear and anxiety related to those memories.
- To re-establish a sense of control by making whatever sense of the trauma they can.
- To re-establish and/or maintain their interpersonal relationships safely.
- Psychotherapy is complex, but controlled evidence is now available that various psychodynamically oriented psychotherapies and cognitive-behavioural therapies are effective.

Future Developments

Predicting the future treatment of anxiety disorders in primary care is difficult because of the problem of knowing whether there will be a ground breaking advance in therapeutics. However, it is my opinion that it is very unlikely that there will be a truly ground breaking change in the medication treatment or psychotherapy of the anxiety disorders in the next 5 years.

Instead, I think that the advances will be primarily in the application of what we largely already know. This will be in terms of increased recognition and better treatment of these disorders with current, but largely under-utilized, treatments. This is particularly true because we have learned in just the last couple years that the SSRI antidepressants are effective in all of the anxiety disorders and are easy to use and well tolerated by patients.

However, this incremental advance in the pharmacotherapy of these conditions is quite important. Even though it has been demonstrated in Western countries, particularly in the US that one SSRI (paroxetine, and probably the other four SSRIs as well), works in all five anxiety disorders, this new advance has not significantly changed clinical practice across the world, even in psychiatry and certainly not in primary care. Not all SSRIs are identical and the next 5–10 years will demonstrate advances and advantages for one SRRI over the others or over current therapies. There are some early suggestions that one SSRI may be more effective in a particular condition than the others.

We will also learn a great deal more about how to use these medications and for what time period. For instance, it is now becoming apparent that the length of treatment needed to maximize the initial response may be as long as 6 months or more. This is particularly true when we are using the appropriate criteria of treating the patient until remission or until they have no symptoms or functional impairments. This will require a significant change in treatment patterns because this is not yet the standard approach in any country. The same set of issues are true for how long these patients should be treated.

One new medication that is on the near horizon is pregabalin, which has been shown to be effective in GAD in the US and may be effective in other anxiety conditions as well. This is a BZ- type drug and, although it is not a BZ, it appears to have many of the advantages of a BZ. Drugs that work on the substance P system and on the corticotropin releasing factor and steroid system are also under active development and show promise. Whether they will offer advances over currently available treatments remains to be seen.

Nonpharmacological somatic treatments are also under active investigation. These include vagal nerve stimulation, in which an intermittent pulse is delivered to the ascending vagal fibres. This is utilized in limited research trials in treatment-resistant anxious patients and shows promise. Similarly, repetitive transcranial magnetic stimulation has shown efficacy in depression and early promise in the anxiety disorders. In this technique, repetitive magnetic pulses to the skull noninvasively affect brain function and is not associated with any side-effects. These and other techniques will evolve to treat the 25–30% of anxiety disorder patients with severe disorders who fail to respond to conventional treatments.

However, an even greater problem remains, i.e. the overwhelming majority of patients who are not recognized and diagnosed, and even when recognized they are not treated adequately. Recognition rates in primary care vary from less than 1% (social anxiety disorder) to 25–50% (PD). My prediction is that as practice and professional organizations and governments realize the cost of not recognizing and treating these patients, changes will evolve, both voluntarily and by direction. For example, in the US, as provider organizations have realized that it is more costly and wasteful not to recognize depression, active attempts are now underway to increase recognition and improve treatments. Some have even involved "top down" approaches, in terms of practice guidelines and standards that are either positively or negatively incentivized. These practices will certainly spread and remains to be seen whether the new Primary Care Trusts or their equivalents in other countries will also incentivize recognition and care of these patients. Patient and public educational efforts are gradually expanding in many countries. For example, it is now clear that efforts to educate members of the public with anxiety disorders (90% of whom never get adequate treatment) can be an effective way for them to learn about, and then assertively seek out their own appropriate treatment.

Other recognition efforts have included attempts to develop questionnaires that can be used by the primary care physician. Many have been developed that are accurate and valid, but generally they require too much time from the physician or his or her staff to be widely accepted. One recent international panel recommended a 10-question screening instrument that would diagnose 95% of the psychiatric conditions in primary care and can be completed by the patient, nurse, or physician in 3–5 minutes.[121] Such an instrument has the promise of being accepted because it might be more widely adopted than other tools that require more time and effort.

So, what does the future hold in improving the medical care of diagnosed anxiety disorder patients in primary care? Surveys of the current situation vary, but still an overwhelming percentage of patients receive treatment that is inadequate for their needs. However, with the likelihood that the SSRIs could become the single treatment for all of these disorders, getting this treatment advance into clinical practice should be easier than most.

However, scientific and treatment advances often take decades or more to become adopted into routine clinical practice. Certainly, particular educational programmes involving the physician, nurse and repeated outreach methods by telephone have been effective in improving the care of depressed patients in primary care and should work for anxiety disorders as well. These have involved collaborative approaches with a psychiatrist offering consultation periodically, in person or by telephone and outreach follow-up. Of the programmes that have been shown to work, it is only those that have a follow-up over weeks and months to ensure that the patient receives the right prescription, fills it, takes the medications, refills the prescriptions, tolerates the side-effects and takes the medicine in appropriate doses and for long enough that have been effective. This type of concerted follow-up is generally done by practice nurses.

If improvements in the care of anxiety disorder patients in primary care are going to occur, it will almost certainly involve programmes that utilize non-physician professionals to provide the support and follow-up necessary for patients to complete the long-term (6–24 months) treatment necessary for recovery from these anxiety disorders.

Frequently Asked Questions

What are anxiety disorders?

Anxiety disorders are the most common of the mental health problems. One in four people will have one or more of the five types of problems (panic, general anxiety, OCD, social anxiety or PTSD).

What is the difference from depression?

Depression is a very different problem with low mood, loss of enjoyment and general tiredness as the main symptoms. Many people with anxiety become depressed as well, often because of the disabling nature of anxiety. It is very common to have mixed anxiety and depression instead of anxiety on its own.

What are the differences between the five types of anxiety?

The different types of anxiety are often easy to spot because of the dominant features of each. Panic anxiety involves PAs, which typically last for up to 20 minutes. Obsessive compulsive anxiety involves the person having specific obsessions (e.g. cleanliness) and compulsions (e.g. hand-washing). Social anxiety involves the person feeling unable to mix in social gatherings. Post trauma anxiety involves being ill after a specific unpleasant occurrence (e.g. being mugged). General anxiety is a mixture of all sorts of anxious thoughts and worries (about everything) other than above with a range of physical symptoms (e.g. tenseness, headache, trouble sleeping).

What is a PA?

PAs are overwhelming periods of extreme anxiety that come out of the blue and reach a peak over around 10 minutes. They then subside usually over a similar period, although people often feel unwell for a few hours. Typical attacks involve feeling the heart pounding fast, trembling and sweating. Many people feel they will die and have to escape from the office, train, restaurant etc. Some people, because of the fear of death, call an ambulance or go to accident and emergency rooms.

Why do I feel anxious between PAs?

This type of anxiety is usually related to the anticipation of further attacks, and the fear of loss of control or even death in the next attack. It often becomes a fear of being in the type of place where it happened before (e.g. being in a crowded train).

Could I die in a PA?

No. The extreme changes in the body are those we all have and use when in a threatening situation (the well known "fight or flight" phenomenon). This type of bodily response has been present and very useful to prevent death (e.g. when chased by dinosaurs!) as it enables us to run away fast or stand and fight.

Why do I have PAs when my diagnosis is PTSD?

PAs can occur in the other anxiety disorders but are different because there is a known and obvious trigger (e.g. thinking about the traumatic event).

I have agoraphobia and PAs. Why is this?

In this situation you have learnt to avoid the situations or places where you have PAs (e.g. trains, shops etc). When severe, some people (around one in 20 with PD) avoid going out of the home altogether. In very extreme cases people can become a recluse and never go out at all unless treated.

How common are PAs?

Around one in 10 of the population have had at least one PA during their lifetime. It is possible to have one or two PAs and never be affected too much or have them again. Some people have them frequently and become ill and most people are between the two extremes of no problem to lots of problems. People are often under some sort of stress when the first attack occurs. They are more common in females in their 20s to 30s.

What causes PAs?

Chemicals in the brain seem to be involved somehow. We know that some of the newer drugs called 'SSRIs' help and this suggests a chemical called serotonin is involved. Much research is being done also on the areas of the brain and the connections or circuits associated with responses to stress.

My GP (or family physician) thought I had a physical problem?

This happens very often because people present to the GP with worrying symptoms that could be physical in origin, such as palpitations, shortness of breath, dizziness etc. Your GP is likely to want to exclude physical causes by arranging tests unless he or she is quite sure that the problem is one of PD or another anxiety disorder. This is often made more likely by people not mentioning their symptoms of anxiety at all or until late in the consultation as most people think their GP is mainly interested in physical problems. It is okay to mention anxieties or worries to your GP at the beginning of a consultation and this may prevent him or her being unnecessarily distracted.

What are the best treatments for PD?

Usually a combination of talking treatments (e.g. supportive listening and a treatment called CBT, which helps you to learn a different way of thinking and responding to PAs and triggering situations) helps with or without medication. The SSRIs seem to be the best medication and are not addictive.

What about BZs?

These drugs can help in the acute situation for a very short time but are not generally prescribed in the longer term because of a risk that some people will take stronger and stronger dosages. Withdrawal should always be gradual to prevent withdrawal symptoms and they should not be taken with alcohol. If used alone there is a possibility that any co-existing depression will not be helped as these drugs are not a treatment for depression.

What is GAD?

This is a persistent increased anxiety and worry about things that might happen (or current events or activities) with the person finding it hard to control the worry. In addition, the person will have at least three or more physical symptoms of muscle tension or worry (e.g. feeling on edge, easily tired, irritable, poor sleep and difficulty concentrating).

How do you tell GAD from depression?

The two problems often occur together and a judgement needs to be made about whether the person is more depressed or anxious. Depression can develop as a result of GAD being present for some time. Some of the symptoms of both are similar (e.g. irritability and fatigue).

How common is GAD?

Eight in every 100 people attending a general practice will have it, and between three and 10 out of every 100 people in the population will get it at some time in their lives. Approximately two out of every three people with GAD will also be depressed or have social anxiety or PD.

Does GAD run in families?

It does run in families and is probably genetic in nature as one in five first-degree relatives will have it (mum, dad, brother, sister etc). It may also be genetically linked to depression in some way.

What are the treatments?

As for other anxiety disorders, either or both of talking treatment or drug treatment seem best. Talking treatment addresses thoughts that are associated with worries and fears (often about failure) and certain associated behaviours (e.g. avoiding situations). General lifestyle factors help, such as cutting down on caffeine, alcohol and cigarettes, and exercise and relaxation often help. There are several possibilities for medication and the pros and cons of each will need to be considered with your doctor.

What is OCD?

OCD consists of obsessions and compulsions. Obsessions are thoughts or images that go round and round in your head and are usually unpleasant and difficult to get rid of. Compulsions are behaviours that are repeated over and over again to try and get rid of the thoughts that will not go. Someone may have recurrent thoughts about being infected by germs and as a result wash dozens of times and still not be convinced. Another common thought might be that "I didn't lock the front door" and the compulsion would be to keep returning to check it.

What is Social Anxiety Disorder?

This is far more than simple shyness and can have a huge negative effect on sufferers. People with this have severe anxiety and fear in social situations. They believe that the people around them will think badly of them and see that they are anxious, nervous, shaky, sweaty etc. People avoid talking to others or doing things in front of others and may develop PAs. Sufferers will not mix with others, eat in front of them or write cheques etc. The person fears being scrutinized by others and that it will be humiliating or embarrassing. Some drink alcohol to reduce these anxieties.

How common is Social Anxiety Disorder?

Very common,with one is six people suffering from it, far higher than originally thought. Most people will have at least one other disorder, such as depression, substance abuse or another anxiety disorder.

What is PTSD?

This is a severe reaction to a traumatic experience whereby the person; relives the trauma (i.e. through flashbacks, nightmares and memories); avoids any triggers (i.e. places) and has exaggerated arousal (i.e. startles easily and irritable).

Does the trauma have to be very extreme like in war-time?

No. Many types of trauma can lead to PTSD, from being raped to having a car accident or seeing someone else suffer a traumatic event. Almost always the event involves a "serious threat to one's life or physical integrity" or to others, family or friends.

A lot of people have traumatic experiences and do not get PTSD?

Yes. In one study half of the men and women in the population had had a traumatic event of some type, yet one in 20 of the men and one in 10 of the women developed PTSD. One in six soldiers in the Vietnam War developed PTSD, with an additional one in 10 having partial PTSD. Approximately, 50–70% of prisoners of war get PTSD and 20–40% of victims of terrorist attacks. Seventy per cent of battered women get PTSD.

References

1. Bridges KW, Goldberg DP. Somatic presentation of DSM III psychiatric disorders in primary care. *J Psychosom Res* 1985; **29**: 563–569.

2. American Psychiatric Association. *Diagnostic and Statistical Manual of Mental Disorders*, 4th Edition. Washington, DC: American Psychiatric Association, 2000.

3. Breier A, Charney DS, Heninger GR. Agoraphobia with panic attacks: development, diagnostic stability, and course of illness. *Arch Gen Psychiatry* 1986; **43**: 1029–1036.

4. Regier DA, Boyd JH, Burke JD *et al*. One-month prevalence of mental disorders in the United States. *Arch Gen Psychiatry* 1988; **45**: 977–986.

5. Kessler RC, McGonagle KA, Zhao S *et al*. Lifetime and 12-month prevalence of DSM III-R psychiatric disorders in the United States: results from the National Comorbidity Survey. *Arch Gen Psychiatry* 1994; **51**: 8–19.

6. Coplan JD, Papp LA, Pine DS *et al*. Clinical improvement with fluoxetine therapy and noradrenergic function in patients with panic disorders. *Arch Gen Psychiatry* 1997; **54**: 643–648.

7. Coplan JD, Gorman JM. Pathogenesis of panic disorder. In: Stein DJ, Hollander E, editors. *Textbook of Anxiety Disorders*. Washington, DC: American Psychiatric Publishing, 2002; pp. 247–256.

8. Ballenger JC. Translational implications of the amygdala-stria terminalis model for the clinical anxiety disorders [editorial]. *Biol Psychiatry* 1998; **44**(12): 1204–1207.

9. Orleans CT, George LK, Houpt JL *et al*. How primary care physicians treat psychiatric disorders: a national survey of family practitioners. *Am J Psychiatry* 1985; **142**: 52–57.

10. Katon W, Vitaliano PP, Russo J *et al*. Panic disorder: epidemiology in primary care. *J Fam Pract* 1986; **23**: 233–239.

11. Lecrubier Y, Ustën TB. Panic and depression: a worldwide primary care perspecive. *Int Clin Psychopharmacol* 1998; **13**(Suppl 4): S7–S11.

12. Simon GE, Von Korff M. Somatization and psychiatric disorders in the NIMH Epidemiologic Catchment Area Study. *Am J Psychiatry* 1991; **148**: 1494–1500.

13. Salvador-Carulla L, Segui J, Fernandez-Cano P *et al*. Costs and offset effect in panic disorders. *Br J Psychiatry* 1995; **166**(Suppl 27): 23–28.

14. Ballenger JC, Davidson JR, Lecrubier Y *et al*. Consensus statement on panic disorder from the International Consensus Group on Depression and Anxiety. *J Clin Psychiatry* 1998; **59**(Suppl 8): 47–54.

15. Gorman JM, Shear MK, McIntyre JS *et al*. Practice guideline for the greatment of patients with panic disorder. *Am J Psychiatry* 1998; **155**(Suppl 5): 1–34.

16. Ballenger JC, Wheadon DE, Steiner M *et al*. Double-blind, fixed-dose, placebo-controlled study of paroxetine in the treatment of panic disorder. *Am J Psychiatry* 1998; **155**(1): 36–42.

17. Pollack MH, Otto MW, Worthington JJ *et al*. Sertraline in the treatment panic disorder: a flexible-dose multi-center trial. *Arch Gen Psychiatry* 1998; **555**: 1010–1016.

18. Michelson D, Lydiard RB, Pollack MH *et al*. Trazodone in the treatment of panic disorder: evidence from a randomized controlled trial of fluoxetine and placebo. The Fluoxetine Panic Disorder Study Group. *Am J Psychiatry* 1998; **155**: 1570–1577.

19. Black DW, Wesner R, Bowers W *et al*. A comparison of fluvoxamine, cognitive therapy and placebo in the treatment of panic disorder. *Arch Gen Psychiatry* 1993; **50**: 44–50.

20. Lepola UM, Wade AG, Leinonen EU *et al*. A controlled, prospective, 1-year trial of citalopram in the treatment of panic disorder. *J Clin Psychiatry* 1998; **59**: 528–534.

21. Boyer W. Serotonin uptake inhibitors are superior to imipramine and alprazolam in alleviating panic attacks: a metanalysis. *Int Clin Psychopharmacol* 1995; **10**: 45–49.

22. Ballenger JC, Burrows G, DuPont RL *et al*. Alprazolam in panic disorder and agoraphobia: results from a multicenter trial. I. Efficacy in short-term treatment. *Arch Gen Psychiatry* 1988; **455**: 413–422.

23. Tesar GE, Rosenbaum JF, Pollack MH *et al*. Double-blind, placebo-controlled comparison of clonazepam and alprazolam for panic disorder. *J. Clin Psychiatry* 1991; **52**: 69–76.

24. Woods SW, Charney DS, Delgado PL *et al*. The effect of long-term imipramine treatment on carbon dioxide-induced anxiety in panic disorder patients. *J Clin Psychiatry* 1990; **51**: 505–507.

25. Uhlenhuth EH, Dwwit H, Balter MB *et al*. Risks and benefits of long-term benzodiazepine use. *J Clin Psychopharmacol* 1988; **8**: 161–167.

26. Ballenger JC. Medication discontinuation in panic disorder. *J Clin Psychiatry* 1992; **53**: 26–31.

27. Otto MW, Pollack MH, Sacks GS *et al*. Discontinuation of benzodiazepine treatment: efficacy of cognitive-behavioral therapy for patients

with panic disorder. *Am J Psychiatry* 1993; **150**: 1485–1490.

28. Lydiard RB, Laraia MT, Ballenger JC *et al.* Emergence of depressive symptoms in patients receiving alprazolam for panic disorder. *J Affect Disord* 1987; **13**: 153–168.

29. Sheehan DV, Ballenger JC, Jacobsen G. Treatment of endogenous anxiety with phobic, hysterical, and hypochondriacal symptoms. *Arch Gen Psychiatry* 1980; **37**: 51–59.

30. DeMartinis NA, Schweizer E, Rickels K. An open-label trial of nefazodone in high comorbidity panic disorder. *J Clin Psychiatry* 1996; **57**: 245–248.

31. Ballenger JC, Davidson JRT, Lecrubier Y *et al.* Consensus statement on generalized anxiety disorder from the International Consensus Group on Depression and Anxiety. *J Clin Psychiatry* 2001; **62**(Suppl 11): 53–58.

32. Cohen LS, Sichel DA, Farone SV *et al.* Course of panic disorder during pregnancy and the puerperium: a preliminary study. *Biol Psychiatry*, 1996; **39**: 950–954.

33. Baum AL, Misri S. Selective serotonin reuptake inhibitors in pregnancy and lactation. *Harv Rev Psychiatry* 1990; **4**: 17–25.

34. Barlow DH, Hofmann SG. Efficacy and dissemination of psychosocial treatment expertise. In: Clark DF, Fairburn CG, editors. *Science and Practice of Cognitive Behaviour Therapy*. Oxford: Oxford University Press, 1997; pp. 95–117.

35. Barlow DH, Craske MG. *Mastery of your Anxiety and Panic*, 2nd Edition (MAPII). Albany: Graywind, 1994.

36. Barlow DH, Craske MG. *Mastery of your Anxiety and Panic*. Albany: Graywind, 1989.

37. Barlow DH, Gorman, JM, Shear MK *et al.* Cognitive-behavioral therapy, imipramine or their combination for panic disorder: a randomized controlled trial. *JAMA* 2000; **283**: 2529–2536.

38. Judd LL, Kessler RC, Paulus HP *et al.* Comorbidity as a fundamental feature of Generalized Anxiety Disorder: results from the National Comorbidity Study (NCS). *Acta Psychiatr Scand Suppl* 1998; **393** : 6–11.

39. Maier W, Falkai P. The epidemiology of comorbidity between depression, anxiety disorders and somatic diseases. *Int Clin Psychopharmacol* 1999; **14**(Suppl 2): S1–S6.

40. Stein DJ. Comorbidity in generalized anxiety disorder: impact and implications. *J Clin Psychiatry* 2001; **62**(Suppl 11): 29–34.

41. Olfson M, Fireman B, Weissman MM *et al.* Mental disorders and disability among patients in primary care practice. *Am J Psychiatry* 1997; **154**: 1734–1740.

42. Ustën TB, Sartorius N. Editors. *Mental Illness in General Health Care: An International Study*. Chichester: John Wiley & Sons, 1995.

43. Goldberg DP, Lecrubier Y. Form and frequency of mental disorders across centers. In: Ustin TB, Sartorius N, editors. *Mental Illness in General Health Care: An International Study*. Chichester: John Wiley & Sons, 1995: pp. 323–334.

44. Wittchen HU, Zahu S, Kessler RC *et al*. DSM-III-R Generalized Anxiety Disorder in the National Comorbidity Survey. *Arch Gen Psychiatry* 1994; **51**: 355–364.

45. Uhlenhuth EH, Balter MB, Mellinger GD *et al*. Symptom Checklist Syndromes in general population: correlations with psychotherapeutic drug use. *Arch Gen Psychiatry* 1983; **40**: 1167–1173.

46. Simonoff E, Pickles A, Myer JM *et al*. The Virginia Twin Study of Adolescent Behavioral Development: influences of age, sex and impairment on rates of disorder. *Arch Gen Psychiatry* 1997; **54**: 801–808.

47. Kendler KS, Neale MC, Kessler RC *et al*. Generalized Anxiety Disorder in women: a population-based twin study. *Arch Gen Psychiatry* 1992; **49**: 267–272.

48. Skre I, Ontad S, Torgersen S *et al*. A twin study of DSMIII-R anxiety disorders. *Acta Psychiatr Scand* 1993; **88**: 85–92.

49. Wu JC, Buchsbaum MS, Hershey TG *et al*. PET in generalized anxiety disorder. *Biol Psychiatry* 1991; **29**: 1181–1199.

50. Aston-Jones G, Rajkowski J, Kubiack P. Conditioned responses among key locus coeruleus neurons anticipate acquisition of discriminative behavior in a vigilance task. *Neuroscience* 1997; **80**: 697–715.

51. Sevy S, Papadimitriou G, Surmont W *et al*. Noradrenergic function in Generalized Anxiety Disorder, Major Depressive Disorder, and healthy subjects. *Biol Psychiatry* 1989; **25**: 141–152.

52. Kahn RS, Wetzler S, Asnis GM *et al*. Pituitary hormone response to meta-chlorophenylpiperazine in panic disorder and health control subjects. *Psychiatry Res 1*991; **37**: 25–34.

53. Weizman R, Tanne Z, Granek M *et al*. Peripheral benzodiazepine binding sites on platelet membranes are increased during diazepam treatment of anxious patients. *Eur J Pharmacol* 1987; **138**: 289–292.

54. Tihonen J, Kuikka J, Rasanen P *et al*. Cerebral benzodiazepine receptor binding and distribution in generalized anxiety disorder: a fractal analysis. *Mol Psychiatry* 1997; **2**: 463–471.

55. Brawman-Mintzer O, Lydiard RB, Villarreal G *et al*. Biological findings in GAD: CCK-B agonist challenge. Paper presented at the 15th National Conference of the Anxiety Disorders Association of America,

Pittsburgh, PA, April 19–21, 1995.

56. Kramer MS, Cutler NR, Ballenger JC *et al*. A placebo-controlled trial of L-365,260 a CCK-B antagonist in panic disorder. *Biol Psychiatry* 1995; **37**(7): 462–466.

57. Lader M. Benzodiazepines: a risk-benefit profile. *CNS Drugs* 1994; **1**: 377–387.

58. Lader MH. Limitations on use of benzodiazepines in anxiety and insomnia: Are they justified? *Eur Psychopharmacol Supp*l 1999; **9**: S399–S405.

59. Argyropulos SV, Nutt DJ. Use of benzodiazepines in anxiety and other disorders. *Eur Neuropsychopharmacol* 1999; (Suppl 6): S407–S412.

60. Ballenger JC. Benzodiazepines. In: Schatzberg AF, Nemeroff CB, editors. *The American Psychiatric Press Textbook of Psychopharmacology*. Washington, DC: American Psychiatric Press, 1995; pp. 215–230.

61. Schweizer E, Rickels K, Uhlenhuth EH. Issues in the long term treatment of anxiety disorders. In: Bloom FE, Kupfer DJ, editors. *Psychopharmacology: The Fourth Generation of Progress*. New York: Raven Press, 1995; pp. 1349–1359.

62. Napoliello MJ. An interim multi-center report on 7,677 anxious geriatric outpatients treated with buspirone. *Br J Clin Pract* 1986; **40**: 71–73.

63. Rakel RE. Long term buspirone therapy for chronic anxiety: a multicenter, international study to determine safety. *South Med J* 1990; **83**: 94–198.

64. Schweizer E, Rickels K, Lucki I. Resistance to the anti-anxiety effects of buspirone in patients with a history of benzodiazepine use. *N Engl J Med* 1986; **314**: 719–720.

65. Gammans RE, Stringfellow JC, Hvizdos AG *et al*. Use of buspirone in patients with Generalized Anxiety Disorder and coexisting depressive symptoms: a meta-analysis of eight randomized, controlled studies. *Neuropsychobiology* 1992; **25**: 193–201.

66. Ferreri M, Hantouche E-G. Recent clinical trials of hydroxyzine in Generalized Anxiety Disorder. *Acta Psychiatr Scand* 1998; **393**: 102–108.

67. Rickels K, Downing R, Schweizer E *et al*. Antidepressants for the treatment of generalized anxiety disorder: a placebo-controlled comparison of imipramine, trazodone, and diazepam. *Arch Gen Psychiatry* 1993; **50**: 884–895.

68. Bellew KM, McCafferty JP, Lyengar M *et al*. Short term efficacy of paroxetine in Generalized Anxiety Disorder: a double-blind, placebo-controlled trial. Presented at the 153rd Annual Meeting of the American

Psychiatric Association, Chicago, May 13–18, 2000 (NR 253).

69. McCafferty, J. Paroxetine is effective in the treatment of generalized anxiety disorder: results from a randomized placebo-controlled flexible-dose study. *Eur Neuropsychopharmacol* 2000; **10**(Suppl 3): S348.

70. Baldwin DS. SSRIs in the treatment of Generalized Anxiety Disorder. SB Satellite Symposium during European College of Neuropsychopharmacology, Munich, 9/10/2000.

71. Borkovec TD, Ruscio AM. Psychotherapy for generalized anxiety disorder. *J Clin Psychiatry* 2001; **62**(Suppl 11): 37–42.

72. Gould RA, Otto MW, Pollack MH *et al*. Cognitive behavioral and pharmacological treatment of Generalized Anxiety Disorder: a preliminary meta-analysis. *Behav Ther* 1997; **28**: 285–305.

73. Durham RC, Fisher PL, Trevling LR *et al*. One year follow up of cognitive therapy, analytical psychotherapy, and anxiety management training for Generalized Anxiety Disorder: symptom change, medication usage, and attitudes to treatment. *Behav Consult Psychother* 1999; **27**: 19–35.

74. Borkovec TD, Abel JL, Newman H. Effects of psychotherapy on comorbid conditions in generalized anxiety disorder. *J Consult Clin Psychol* 1995; **63**: 479–483.

75. Mynors-Wallis L, Gath D. Predictors for treatment outcome for major depression in primary care. *Psychol Med* 1997; **27**: 731–736.

76. Lader MH, Bond AG. Interaction of pharmacological and psychological treatments of anxiety. *Br J Psychiatry* 1998; **173**(Suppl 34): 42–48.

77. Wardle J. Behavior therapy and benzodiazepines: allies or antagonists? *Br J Psychiatry* 1990; **156**: 163–168.

78. Power KG, Simpson RJ, Swanson V *et al*. A controlled cognitive behavioral therapy, diazepam and placebo, alone and in combination, for the treatment of Generalized Anxiety Disorder. *J Anxiety Disorder* 1990; **4**: 267–292.

79. Stein AJ, Hollander E. Editors. *Textbook of Anxiety Disorders*. Washington DC: American Psychiatric Publishing, 2002.

80. MacDougle CJ, Goodman WK, Leckman JF *et al*. Haloperidal addition to fluvoxamine – refractory Obsessive Compulsive Disorder: a double blind, placebo-controlled study in patients with and without tics. *Arch Gen Psychiatry* 1994; **51**: 302–308.

81. Robbins LN, Helzer JF, Weissman MM *et al*. Lifetime prevalence of specific psychiatric disorders in three sites. *Arch Gen Psychiatry* 1984; **41**: 958–967.

82. Apter A, Fallon TJ, King RA *et al*. Obsessive compulsive characteristics: from symptoms to syndrome. *J Am Acad Child Adoles Psychiatry* 1996; **35**: 907–912.

83. Pauls BL, Alsobrook JP, Goodman W *et al*. A family study of Obsessive Compulsive Disorder. *Am J Psychiatry* 1995; **152**: 76–84.

84. Swedo SE, Leonard HL, Garvey M *et al*. Paediatric Autoimmune Neuropsychiatric Disorders Associated with Streptococcus Infection (PANDAS): clinical description of the first 50 cases. *Am J Psychiatry* 1998; **155**: 264–271.

85. Rasmussen SA, Eisen JL. The epidemiology and clinical features of Obsessive Compulsive Disorder. In: Jenike MA, Baer L, Minichiello WE, editors. *Obsessive Compulsive Disorders: Practical Management*, 3rd Edition. St. Louis: Mosby, 1998; pp. 12–43.

86. Demal U, Gerhardt L, Mayrhofer A *et al*. Obsessive Compulsive Disorder and depression. *Psychopathology* 1993; **26**: 145–150.

87. Pato NT, Hill JL, Murphy DL. A clomipramine dose reduction study in the course of long-term treatment of Obsessive Compulsive Disorder patients. *Psychopharmacol Bull* 1990; **26**: 211–214.

88. Ravizza L, Barzega G, Bellino S *et al*. Drug treatment of OCD: long-term trial with clomipramine and selective serotonin reuptake inhibitors (SSRIs). *Psychopharmacol Bull* 1996; **32**: 167–173.

89. Marks IM, Baer L, Greist JH *et al*. Home self-assessment of Obsessive-Compulsive Disorder: use of a manual and a computer-conducted telephone interview. Two UK-US studies. *Br J Psychiatry* 1998; **172**: 406–412.

90. Stein MD, Fyer AJ, Davidson JRT *et al*. Fluvoxamine treatment of social phobia (social anxiety disorder): a double-blind, placebo-controlled study. *Am J Psychiatry* 1999; **156**: 756–760.

91. Wyler E, Bisserbe JC, Boyer P *et al*. Social phobia in the general health care: An unrecognized and treated disabling disorder. G*en Psychiatry* 1996; **168**: 169–174.

92. Fyer AJ, Mannuzza S, Chapman TE *et al*. A direct interview family study of social phobia. *Arch Gen Psychiatry* 1993; **50**: 286–293.

93. Stein MD, Chartier MJ, Hazen AL *et al*. A direct interview family study of generalized social phobia. *Med J Psychiatry* 1998; **155**: 90–97.

94. Kendler KS, Neale MC, Kupford RC *et al*. The genetic epidemiology of phobias in women: an interrelationship of agoraphobia, social phobia, situational phobia, and simple phobia. *Arch Gen Psychiatry* 1992; **49**: 273–281.

95. Tihonen J, Kuikka JA, Bergstrom K *et al*. Dopamine reuptake site densities in patients with social phobia. *Am J Psychiatry* 1997; 154: 239–242.

96. Stein MD, Chartier MJ, Hazen AL *et al*. Paroxetine in the treatment of generalized social phobia: open-label treatment and double-blind placebo-controlled discontinuation. *J Clin Psychopharmacol* 1996; **16**: 218–222.

97. van Vliet IM, den Boer JA, Westenberg HG. Psychopharmacological treatment of social phobia: a double-blind placebo-controlled study with fluvoxamine. *Psychopharmacology* 1994; **115**: 128–134.

98. Davidson JRT, Postie LS, Richichi E *et al*. Treatment of social phobia with clonazepam and placebo. *J Clin Psychopharmacol* 1993; **13**: 423–428.

99. Gelernter CS, Uhde TW, Cimbolic P *et al*. Cognitive-behavioral and pharmacological treatments of social phobia: a controlled study. *Arch Gen Psychiatry* 1991; **48**: 938.

100. Liebowitz MR, Schneier FR, Campeas R *et al*. Phenelzine versus atenolol in social phobia: a placebo-controlled comparison. *Arch Gen Psychiatry* 1992; **49**: 290–300.

101. Fahlen T, Nilsson HL, Humble M *et al*. Social phobia: The clinical efficacy and tolerability of the monoamine oxidase A and serotonin reuptake inhibitor brofaromine: a double-blind placebo-controlled study. *Acta Psychiatr Scand* 1995; **92**: 351–358.

102. Lott M, Greist JH, Jefferson JW *et al*. Brofaromine for social phobia: a multicenter, placebo-controlled, double-blind study. *J Clin Psychopharmacol* 1997; **17**: 255–260.

103. Versiani M, Nardi AE, Mundim FD *et al*. Pharmacotherapy of social phobia: a controlled study with moclobemide and phenelzine. *Br J Psychiatry* 1992; **161**: 353–360.

104. Turner SM, Beidel DC, Jacob RG. Social phobia: a comparison of behavior therapy and atenolol. *J Consult Clin Psychol* 1994; 62: 350–358.

105. Ballenger JC, Davidson JRT, Lecrubier Y *et al*. Consensus statement on social anxiety disorder from the International Consensus Group on Depression and Anxiety. *J Clin Psychiatry* 1998; **59**(Suppl 17); 54–60.

106. Heimberg RG, Juster HR. Cognitive-behavioral treatments: Literature review. In: Heimberg RG, Liebowitz MR, Hope DA *et al*., editors. *Social Phobia: Diagnosis, Assessment, and Treatment*. New York: Guilford Press, 1995; pp. 261–309.

107. Turner SM, Beidel DC, Cooley-Quille MR. Two-year follow-up study of social phobics treated with social effectiveness therapy. *Behav Res Ther* 1995; **33**: 553–555.

108. Heimberg RG, Liebowitz MR, Hope DA *et al*. Cognitive-behav-

ioral group therapy versus phenelzine in social phobia: 12-week outcome. *Arch Gen Psychiatry* 1998; **55**: 1133–1141.

109. Lipsitz JD, Markowitz JC, Cherry S *et al*. Open trial of interpersonal psychotherapy for the treatment of social phobia. *Am J Psychiatry* 1999; **156**: 1814–1816.

110. Breslau N, Davis GC, Andreski P *et al*. Traumatic stress disorder in urban populations of young adults. *Arch Gen Psychiatry* 1991; **48**: 216–222.

111. Kessler RC, Sonnega A, Bromet E *et al*. Post-traumatic stress disorder in the National Comorbidity Survey. *Arch Gen Psychiatry* 1995; **52**: 1048–1060.

112. Kulka AR, Schlenger WE, Fairbank JA. Trauma and the Vietnam War Generation: report of the Findings from the National Vietnam Veterans Readjustment Study. New York: Brunner/Mazel, 1990.

113. Yehuda R, Siever L, Teicher MH *et al*. Plasma norepinephrine and MHPG-concentrations and severity of depression in combat PTSD and major depressive disorder. *Biol Psychiatry* 1998; **44**: 56–63.

114. Resnick HS, Yehuda R, Pittman RK *et al*. Effect of previous trauma on acute plasma cortisol level following rape. *Am J Psychiatry* 1995; **152**: 1675–1677.

115. McFarlane AC, Atchison M, Yehuda R. The acute stress response following motor vehicle accidents and its relationship to PTSD. *Ann NY Acad Sci* 1997; **821**: 437–441.

116. Shalev AY, Sahar T, Freedman S *et al*. A prospective study of heart rate response following trauma and the subsequent development of post-traumatic stress disorder. *Arch Gen Psychiatry* 1998; **55**: 553–559.

117. McEwen BS. Protective and damaging effects of stress-mediated. *New Engl J Med* 1998; **338**: 171–179.

118. Marshall RD, Beebe KL, Oldham M *et al*. Efficacy and safety of paroxetine treatment for chronic PTSD: a fixed-dose, placebo-controlled study. *Am J Psychiatry* 2001; **158**(12): 1982–1988.

119. Davidson JRT, Weisler RH, Malik ML *et al*. Treatment of post-traumatic stress disorder with nefazodone. *Int Clin Psychopharmacol* 1998; **13**: 111–113.

120. Davidson JRT, Kudler HS, Smith R *et al*. Treatment of post-traumatic stress disorder with amitriptyline and placebo. *Arch Gen Psychiatry*, 1990; **47**: 259–266.

121. Ballenger JC, Davidson JRT, Lecrubier Y *et al*. A proposed algorithm for improved recognition and treatment of the depression/anxiety spectrum in primary care. *Primary Care Companion J Clin Psychiatry* 2001; **3**: 44–52.

Appendix 1 – Drugs

Drug	Trade name	Preparation	Strength	Doses used in anxiety disorders (adult)	Comments	Side-effects
Anxiolytics						
Alprazolam	Xanax	Tablet	0.25 mg, 0.5 mg, 1 mg*, 2 mg*	Short-term treatment of anxiety: 0.25–0.5 mg 3 times/day (elderly or debilitated, renal and hepatic impairment 0.25 mg 3 times/day) (max 3 mg/day). Up to 10mg/d in PD	Contraindicated in respiratory depression, acute pulmonary insufficiency, sleep apnoea syndrome, phobic and obsessional states, chronic psychosis (not in US), severe hepatic impairment; caution in respiratory disease, muscle weakness, history of drug/alcohol abuse, avoid prolonged use and abrupt withdrawal	Drowsiness, confusion, ataxia (especially elderly), dependence, paradoxical increase in aggression, muscle weakness
Chlor-diazepoxide	Librium	Capsule	5 mg, 10 mg, 25 mg*	Short-term treatment of anxiety: 10 mg 3 times/day; elderly or debilitated, hepatic and renal impairment half adult dose	Indicated in short-term treatment of anxiety; contraindicated in respiratory depression, acute pulmonary insufficiency, sleep apnoea syndrome, phobic and obsessional states, chronic psychosis, severe hepatic impairment; caution in respiratory disease, muscle weakness, history of drug/alcohol abuse, avoid prolonged use and abrupt withdrawal	Drowsiness, confusion, ataxia (especially elderly), dependence, paradoxical increase in aggression, muscle weakness, sedation if used with alcohol
		Powder for injection*	100 mg*			

* Only available in US

Drug	Trade name	Preparation	Strength	Doses used in anxiety disorders (adult)	Comments	Side-effects
Anxiolytics						
Clorazepate	Tranxene	Capsule	3.75 mg* 7.5 mg 15 mg	Short-term treatment of anxiety: 7.5–22.5 mg/day in 2–3 divided doses, elderly or debilitated, hepatic and renal impairment half adult dose	Contraindicated in respiratory depression, acute pulmonary insufficiency, sleep apnoea syndrome, phobic and obsessional states, chronic psychosis (not in US), severe hepatic impairment; caution in respiratory disease, muscle weakness, history of drug/alcohol abuse, avoid prolonged use and abrupt withdrawal	Drowsiness, confusion, ataxia (especially elderly), dependence, paradoxical increase in aggression, muscle weakness, sedation if used with alcohol
		Tablets*	3.75 mg*, 7.5 mg,* 11.25 mg,* 15 mg,* 22.5 mg*			
Diazepam	Valium	Tablet	2 mg, 5 mg, 10 mg	Short-term treatment of anxiety 2 mg 3 times/day increasing to 15–30 mg/day in divided doses prn, elderly or debilitated, hepatic and renal impairment half adult dose	Contraindicated in respiratory depression, acute pulmonary insufficiency, sleep apnoea syndrome, phobic and obsessional states, chronic psychosis (not in US), severe hepatic impairment; caution in respiratory disease, muscle weakness, history of drug/alcohol abuse, avoid prolonged use and abrupt withdrawal; I/M and slow I/V injection used for severe anxiety and acute PAs and status epilepticus*	Drowsiness, confusion, ataxia (especially elderly), dependence, paradoxical increase in aggression, muscle weakness
	Valium	Oral solution	2 mg/ml 5 mg/ml			
	Valium	Injection	5 mg/ml*	10 mg every 4 hours prn		
	Stesolid	Rectal tubes	5 mg, 10 mg, 15 mg,* 20 mg*	500 mcg/kg every 12 hours prn (elderly 250 mcg)		

* Only available in US

Drug	Trade name	Preparation	Strength	Doses used in anxiety disorders (adult)	Comments	Side-effects
Anxiolytics						
Lorazepam	Ativan	Tablet	1 mg, 2.5 mg	Short-term treatment of anxiety: 1–4 mg/day in divided doses, elderly or debilitated, hepatic and renal impairment half adult dose.	Contraindicated in respiratory depression, acute pulmonary insufficiency, sleep apnoea syndrome, phobic and obsessional states, chronic psychosis (not in US), severe hepatic impairment; caution in respiratory disease, muscle weakness, history of drug/alcohol abuse, avoid prolonged use and abrupt withdrawal; I/M and slow I/V injection used for acute PAs; or manic excitement*; short acting	Drowsiness, confusion, ataxia (especially elderly), dependence, paradoxical increase in aggression, muscle weakness, sedation if used with alcohol
	Ativan	Injection	4 mg/ml	25–30 mcg/kg every 6 hours prn		
Oxazepam	Generic	Tablet	10 mg, 15 mg, 30 mg	Short-term treatment of anxiety: 15–30 mg (elderly or debilitated, hepatic and renal impairment 10–20 mg) 3–4 times/day	Contraindicated in respiratory depression, acute pulmonary insufficiency, sleep apnoea syndrome, phobic and obsessional states, chronic psychosis (not in US), severe hepatic impairment; caution in respiratory disease, muscle weakness, history of drug/alcohol abuse, avoid prolonged use and abrupt withdrawal; short acting	Drowsiness, confusion, ataxia (especially elderly), dependence, paradoxical increase in aggression, muscle weakness, sedation if used with alcohol
	Serax*	Capsule	15 mg,* 10 mg,* 30 mg*			

* Only available in US

Drug	Trade name	Preparation	Strength	Doses used in anxiety disorders (adult)	Comments	Side-effects
Anxiolytics						
Buspirone	Buspar	Tablet	5 mg, 10 mg, 15 mg*	Short-term treatment of anxiety: 5 mg 2–3 times/day. range 15–30 mg/day in divided doses (max 45 mg)	Indicated in short-term treatment of anxiety (low dependence potential but response may take up to 2 weeks); contraindicated in epilepsy, severe hepatic or renal impairment, pregnancy and breastfeeding	Nausea, dizziness, headache, nervousness, light-headedness, excitement
Beta-adrenoceptor blocking drugs (not available in US)						
Oxprenolol	Trasicor	Tablet	20 mg, 40 mg, 80 mg	Short-term treatment of anxiety: 40–80 mg/day	Most suitable for patients with palpitations, tremor or tachycardia; contraindicated in asthma or obstructive airways disease, uncontrolled heart failure, hypotension; caution in pregnancy and breastfeeding, hepatic and renal impairment (reduce dose)	Bradycardia, heart failure, hypotension, conduction disorders, bronchospasm, peripheral vasoconstriction, gastrointestinal effects, fatigue, sleep disturbances
Propranolol	Inderal	Tablet	10 mg, 40 mg, 80 mg	Short-term treatment of anxiety: 40–120 mg/day	Most suitable for patients with palpitations, tremor or tachycardia; contraindicated in asthma or obstructive airways disease, uncontrolled heart failure, hypotension; caution in pregnancy and breastfeeding	Bradycardia, heart failure, hypotension, conduction disorders, bronchospasm, peripheral vasoconstriction, gastrointestinal effects, fatigue, sleep disturbances

* Only available in US

Drug	Trade name	Preparation	Strength	Doses used in anxiety disorders (adult)	Comments	Side-effects
Antipsychotic drugs (not available in US)						
Chlorpromazine	Largactil	Tablet Syrup Suspension forte Injection	10 mg, 25 mg, 50 mg, 100 mg 25 mg/5 ml 100 mg/5 ml 25 mg/ml	Short-term treatment of severe anxiety: 25 mg 3 times/day. elderly or debilitated one-third to half adult dose 25–50 mg every 6–8 hours	Contraindicated in coma caused by CNS depressants; bone marrow depression; caution in cardiovascular or cerebrovascular disease, epilepsy, renal and hepatic impairment, pregnancy and breastfeeding, hypothyroidism, glaucoma; deep I/M injection used to control acute symptoms; avoid direct exposure to sun	Extrapyramidal symptoms (reversed by dose reduction and antimuscarinic agents), hypothermia, drowsiness, apathy, pallor, nightmares, depression, antimuscarinic symptoms (dry mouth, constipation, difficulty with micturition, blurred vision), cardiovascular symptoms (hypotension, tachycardia, arrhythmias), respiratory depression, impotence, sensitivity reactions (blood, photosensitivity, rashes), neuroleptic malignant syndrome
Fluphenazine	Moditen	Tablet	1 mg, 2.5 mg, 5 mg	Short-term treatment of severe anxiety: 1 mg 2 times/day increasing to 2 mg 2 times/day prn	Contraindicated in coma caused by CNS depressants, bone marrow depression; caution in cardiovascular or cerebrovascular disease, epilepsy, renal and hepatic impairment, pregnancy and breastfeeding, hypothyroidism, glaucoma	Extrapyramidal symptoms (more frequent than chlorpromazine – reversed by dose reduction and antimuscarinic agents), hypothermia, drowsiness (less sedating than chlorpromazine), apathy, pallor, nightmares, depression, antimuscarinic symptoms (less frequent than chlorpromazine – dry mouth, constipation, difficulty with micturition, blurred vision), cardiovascular symptoms (hypotension, tachycardia, arrhythmias), respiratory depression, impotence, sensitivity reactions (blood, photosensitivity, rashes), neuroleptic malignant syndrome

Drug	Trade name	Preparation	Strength	Doses used in anxiety disorders (adult)	Comments	Side-effects
Antipsychotic drugs (not available in US)						
Haloperidol	Haldol	Tablet Oral liquid Injection Capsule	5 mg, 10 mg 2 mg/ml 5 mg/ml 500 mcg	Short-term treatment of severe anxiety: 500 mcg 2 times/day	Contraindicated in coma caused by CNS depressants, bone marrow depression, basal ganglia disease; caution in cardiovascular or cerebrovascular disease, epilepsy, renal and hepatic impairment, pregnancy and breastfeeding, hypothyroidism, glaucoma; deep I/M injection used to control acute symptoms	Extrapyramidal symptoms (more frequent than chlorpromazine – reversed by dose reduction and antimuscarinic agents), hypothermia, drowsiness (less sedating than chlorpromazine), apathy, pallor, nightmares, depression, antimuscarinic symptoms (less frequent than chlorpromazine – dry mouth, constipation, difficulty with micturition, blurred vision), cardiovascular symptoms (hypotension, tachycardia, arrhythmias), respiratory depression, impotence, sensitivity reactions (blood, rashes), neuroleptic malignant syndrome
	Serenace	Tablet Oral liquid Injection	1.5 mg, 5 mg, 10 mg 2 mg/ml 5 mg/ml, 10 mg/ml			
Oxypertine	Oxypertine	Capsule	10 mg	Short-term treatment of severe anxiety: 10 mg 3–4 times/day (max 60 mg/day)	Contraindicated in coma caused by CNS depressants, bone marrow depression; caution in cardiovascular or cerebrovascular disease, epilepsy, renal and hepatic impairment, pregnancy and breastfeeding, hypothyroidism, glaucoma	Extrapyramidal symptoms (less frequent than chlorpromazine – reversed by dose reduction and antimuscarinic agents), hypothermia, drowsiness, apathy, pallor, nightmares, depression, antimuscarinic symptoms (dry mouth, constipation, difficulty with micturition, blurred vision), cardiovascular symptoms (hypotension, tachycardia, arrhythmias), respiratory depression, impotence, sensitivity reactions (blood, photosensitivity, rashes), neuroleptic malignant syndrome

Drug	Trade name	Preparation	Strength	Doses used in anxiety disorders (adult)	Comments	Side-effects
Antipsychotic drugs (not available in US)						
Pericyazine	Neulactil	Tablet Syrup	2.5 mg, 10 mg 10 mg/5 ml	Short-term treatment of severe anxiety: 15–30 mg/day (elderly 5–10 mg/day) in 2 divided doses	Contraindicated in coma caused by CNS depressants, bone marrow depression; caution in cardiovascular or cerebrovascular disease, epilepsy, renal and hepatic impairment, pregnancy and breastfeeding, hypothyroidism, glaucoma	Extrapyramidal symptoms (reversed by dose reduction and antimuscarinic agents), hyperthermia, drowsiness (more sedating than chlorpromazine), apathy, pallor, nightmares, depression, antimuscarinic symptoms (dry mouth, constipation, difficulty with micturition, blurred vision), cardiovascular symptoms (hypotension, tachycardia, arrhythmias), respiratory depression, impotence, sensitivity reactions (blood, photosensitivity, rashes), neuroleptic malignant syndrome
Perphenazine	Fentazin	Tablet	2 mg, 4 mg	Short-term treatment of severe anxiety: 4 mg 3 times/day (max 24 mg); elderly quarter to half adult dose	Contraindicated in coma caused by CNS depressants, bone marrow depression; caution in cardiovascular or cerebrovascular disease, epilepsy, renal and hepatic impairment, pregnancy and breastfeeding, hypothyroidism, glaucoma	Extrapyramidal symptoms (more frequent than chlorpromazine – reversed by dose reduction and antimuscarinic agents), hypothermia, drowsiness (less sedating than chlorpromazine), apathy, pallor, nightmares, depression, antimuscarinic symptoms (dry mouth, constipation, difficulty with micturition, blurred vision), cardiovascular symptoms (hypotension, tachycardia, arrhythmias), respiratory depression, endocrine effects, impotence, sensitivity reactions (blood, photosensitivity, rashes), neuroleptic malignant syndrome

Drug	Trade name	Preparation	Strength	Doses used in anxiety disorders (adult)	Comments	Side-effects
Antipsychotic drugs (not available in US)						
Prochlor-perazine	Stemetil	Tablet Syrup	5 mg. 25 mg. 5 mg/5 ml	Short-term treatment of severe anxiety: 15–20 mg/day in divided doses (max 40 mg/day)	Contraindicated in coma caused by CNS depressants, bone marrow depression; caution in cardiovascular or cerebrovascular disease, epilepsy, renal and hepatic impairment, pregnancy and breastfeeding, hypothyroidism, glaucoma	Extrapyramidal symptoms (more frequent than chlorpromazine – reversed by dose reduction and antimuscarinic agents), tardive dyskinesia (prolonged administration), hypothermia, drowsiness (less sedating than chlorpromazine), apathy, pallor, nightmares, depression, antimuscarinic symptoms (dry mouth, constipation, difficulty with micturition, blurred vision), cardiovascular symptoms (hypotension, tachycardia, arrhythmias), respiratory depression, impotence, sensitivity reactions (blood, photosensitivity, rashes), neuroleptic malignant syndrome, corneal and lens opacities and skin pigmentation (prolonged administration)

Drug	Trade name	Preparation	Strength	Doses used in anxiety disorders (adult)	Comments	Side-effects
Antipsychotic drugs (not available in US)						
Trifluoperazine	Stelazine	Tablet M/R capsule Syrup	1 mg, 5 mg, 2 mg, 10 mg, 15 mg 1 mg/5 ml	Short-term treatment of severe anxiety: 2–4 mg/day (max 6 mg/day)	Contraindicated in coma caused by CNS depressants, bone marrow depression; caution in cardiovascular or cerebrovascular disease, epilepsy, renal and hepatic impairment, pregnancy and breastfeeding, hypothyroidism, glaucoma; M/R formulation should be swallowed whole	Extrapyramidal symptoms (more frequent than chlorpromazine – reversed by dose reduction and antimuscarinic agents), hypothermia, drowsiness (less sedating than chlorpromazine), apathy, pallor, nightmares, depression, antimuscarinic symptoms (less frequent than chlorpromazine – dry mouth, constipation, difficulty with micturition, blurred vision), cardiovascular symptoms (hypotension, tachycardia, arrhythmias), respiratory depression, impotence, sensitivity reactions (blood, photosensitivity, rashes), neuroleptic malignant syndrome
Tricyclic antidepressant drugs						
Clomipramine	Anafranil	Capsule	10 mg, 25 mg, 50 mg, 75 mg*	Obsessional states and social phobia: 25 mg/day (elderly 10 mg/day), maintenance: 100–150 mg/day	Contraindicated in recent myocardial infarction, arrhythmias, severe hepatic impairment; caution in cardiac disease, history of epilepsy, pregnancy and breastfeeding, thyroid disease, psychoses, glaucoma, urinary retention	Dry mouth, sedation, blurred vision, constipation, nausea, difficulty with micturition, cardiovascular effects (arrhythmias, postural hypotension, syncope, tachycardia), hypersensitivity reactions, mania, weight change, movement disorders, fever, agranulocytosis

Tricyclic antidepressant drugs

Drug	Trade name	Preparation	Strength	Doses used in anxiety disorders (adult)	Comments	Side-effects
Imipramine*	Tofranil	Capsule	75 mg,* 100 mg,* 125 mg,* 150 mg*		Contraindicated in recent myocardial infarction, arrhythmias, severe hepatic impairment; caution in cardiac disease, history of epilepsy, pregnancy and breastfeeding, thyroid disease, psychoses, glaucoma, urinary retention	Dry mouth, sedation, blurred vision, constipation, nausea, difficulty with micturition, cardiovascular effects (arrhythmias, postural hypotension, syncope, tachycardia), hypersensitivity reactions, mania, weight change, movement disorders, fever, agranulocytosis
		Tablet	10 mg,* 25 mg, 50 mg*			
		Injection	12.5 mg/ml*			

* Only available in US

Drug	Trade name	Preparation	Strength	Doses used in anxiety disorders (adult)	Comments	Side-effects
Reversible MAOIs (not available in US)						
Moclobemide	Manerix	Tablet	150 mg, 300 mg	Social phobia: 300 mg/day increasing to 300 mg 2 times/day on day 4	Treat for 8–12 weeks to assess efficacy; contraindicated in acute confusional states, phaeochromocytoma; caution in agitated patients, thyrotoxicosis, pregnancy and breastfeeding; hepatic impairment	Sleep disturbances, dizziness, gastrointestinal effects, headache, restlessness, agitation, paraesthesia, dry mouth, visual disturbances, oedema, skin reactions, confusional states
SSRIs						
Citalopram	Cipramil Celexa*	Tablet	10 mg, 20 mg, 40 mg	PD: 10 mg/day increasing to 20 mg/day on day 4, range 20–30 mg/day (max 60 mg/day. elderly 40 mg/day)	Caution in epilepsy, history of mania, cardiac disease, history of bleeding disorders, renal and hepatic impairment (reduce dose), pregnancy and breastfeeding; avoid abrupt withdrawal	Gastrointestinal effects (nausea, vomiting, dyspepsia, abdominal pain, diarrhoea, constipation), anorexia, weight changes, hypersensitivity reactions, palpitations, tachycardia, postural hypotension, coughing, confusion, impaired concentration, amnesia, migraine, sedation with alcohol
		Oral drops	40 mg/ml			
Escitalopram	Cipralex Lexapro*	Tablet	10 mg	PD: 5 mg/day increasing to 10 mg/day on day 7 (max 20 mg/day); use lower doses in elderly	Caution in epilepsy, history of mania, cardiac disease, history of bleeding disorders, renal and hepatic impairment (reduce dose); pregnancy and breastfeeding; avoid abrupt withdrawal	Gastrointestinal effects (nausea, vomiting, dyspepsia, abdominal pain, diarrhoea, constipation), anorexia, weight changes, hypersensitivity reactions, palpitations, tachycardia, postural hypotension, impaired concentration, amnesia, migraine

* Only available in US

Drug	Trade name	Preparation	Strength	Doses used in anxiety disorders (adult)	Comments	Side-effects
SSRIs						
Fluoxetine	Prozac	Capsule Liquid	10 mg,* 20 mg, 60 mg 20 mg/5 ml	OCD: 20 mg/day for several weeks (max 60 mg/day)	Caution in epilepsy, history of mania, cardiac disease, history of bleeding disorders, renal and hepatic impairment (reduce dose), pregnancy and breastfeeding; avoid abrupt withdrawal	Gastrointestinal effects (nausea, vomiting, dyspepsia, abdominal pain, diarrhoea, constipation), anorexia, weight loss, hypersensitivity reactions (angioedema, urticaria, anaphylaxis - discontinue if rash occurs), changes in blood sugar, fever, neuroleptic malignant syndrome like event
Fluvoxamine	Faverin Luvox*	Tablet	50 mg, 100 mg	OCD: 100 mg/day (max 300 mg/day)	Treat for 10 weeks to assess response; caution in epilepsy, history of mania, cardiac disease, history of bleeding disorders, renal and hepatic impairment (reduce dose), pregnancy and breastfeeding; avoid abrupt withdrawal	Gastrointestinal effects (nausea, vomiting, dyspepsia, abdominal pain, diarrhoea, constipation), anorexia, weight loss, hypersensitivity reactions (rash, pruritus, arthralgia, myalgia, photosensitivity, anaphylactoid reactions), palpitations, tachycardia, confusion, increases levels of BZs

* Only available in US

Drug	Trade name	Preparation	Strength	Doses used in anxiety disorders (adult)	Comments	Side-effects
SSRIs						
Paroxetine	Seroxat Paxil*	Tablet Liquid	12mg*, 20 mg, 30 mg, 40 mg* 10 mg/5 ml	OCD: 20 mg/day. (max 60 mg/day): PD: 10 mg/day (40 mg/day*), (max 50 mg/day); social phobia: 20 mg/day (max 50 mg/day); GAD 20 mg/day; PTSD 20 mg/day (max 50 mg/day)	Panic symptoms may worsen during initial treatment for PD; caution in epilepsy, history of mania, cardiac disease, history of bleeding disorders, elderly, renal and hepatic impairment (reduce dose), pregnancy and breastfeeding; avoid abrupt withdrawal (withdrawal syndrome reported)	Gastrointestinal effects (nausea, vomiting, dyspepsia, abdominal pain, diarrhoea, constipation), anorexia, weight loss, hypersensitivity reactions (rash, urticaria, pruritus, angioedema), extrapyramidal effects (including orofacial dystonias), postural hypotension
Sertraline	Lustral Zoloft*	Tablet	25mg*, 50 mg, 100 mg	OCD: start 50 mg/day, increase by 50mg/day increments. Max dose 200 mg/day	Caution in epilepsy, history of mania, cardiac disease, history of bleeding disorders, renal and hepatic impairment (reduce dose), pregnancy and breastfeeding; avoid abrupt withdrawal	Gastrointestinal effects (nausea, vomiting, dyspepsia, abdominal pain, diarrhoea, constipation), anorexia, weight loss, hypersensitivity reactions (rash, erythema multiforme, photosensitivity, angioedema, arthralgia, myalgia), tachycardia, confusion, amnesia, hallucinations, aggressive behaviour, psychosis, pancreatitis, hepatitis, jaundice

* Only available in US

Drug	Trade name	Preparation	Strength	Doses used in anxiety disorders (adult)	Comments	Side-effects
Irreversible MAOIs						
Phenelzine	Nardil	Tablet	15 mg	30–45 mg/day Max dose 60 mg/day)	Treat for 6–12 weeks to assess efficacy. Used particularly in PD and social phobia	Tachycardia, palpiations, muscle twitching, seizures, insomnia, transient hypertension, hyperplexia, sedation with alcohol, avoid tyramine containing foods
Tranylcy-promine	Parnate	Tablet	10 mg	10 mg 2 times/d increase by 10 mg increments at 1–3 week intervals. max. 60 mg/d	Avoid food high in tyramine, increased onset of therapeutic effect more than other MAOIs causes more severe hypertensive reactions. Contraindicated in uncontrolled hypertension, pheochromocytoma, cardiovascular disease, renal or hepatic impairment.	Drowsiness, hyperexcitability, headaches, dry mouth, constipation, urinary retention, blurred vision, hepatitis, photosensitivity, rash, orthostatic hypotension

Drug	Trade name	Preparation	Strength	Doses used in anxiety disorders (adult)	Comments	Side-effects
Other antidepressant drugs						
Venlafaxine	Efexor Effexor*	Tablet	25 mg,* 37.5 mg,* 50 mg,* 75 mg,* 100 mg,* 150 mg	GAD: 75 mg/day, 75–200 mg/d* (max 300–350 mg/d)	Treat for 8 weeks to assess response; contraindicated in severe renal and hepatic impairment, pregnancy and breastfeeding; caution in history of myocardial infarction, history of epilepsy, avoid abrupt withdrawal	Nausea, headache, insomnia, somnolence, dry mouth, dizziness, constipation, asthenia, sweating, nervousness, convulsions, increases in blood pressure at higher doses (>300 mg/d)
	Efexor XL Effexor XL*	Capsule	75 mg, 150 mg			

* Only available in US

Appendix 2 — Useful Addresses and Websites

Anxiety Care
Cardinal Heenan Centre
326 High Road
Ilford
Essex IG1 1QP
United Kingdom
Tel: +44 (0)20 8262 8891/2
Web: http://www.anxietycare.org.uk

Anxiety Disorders Association of America
8730 Georgia Avenue, Suite 600
Silver Spring
MD 20910, USA
Tel: 1 240 485 1001
Fax: 1 240 485 1035
Website: http://www.adaa.org/

American Mental Health Resources, Inc
21 Bloomingdale Road
White Plains, NY 10605, USA
Website: http://www.amhronline.com

American Psychiatric Association
1400 K Street NW,
Washington,
DC 20005, USA
Tel: (888) 357 7924
Fax: 1 202 682 6850
Website: http://www.psych.org/index.cfm

Freedom from Fear
308 Seaview Avenue,
Staten Island

NY 10305, USA
Tel: 1 888 442 2022
Website: http://www.freedomfromfear.com

National Anxiety Foundation
3135 Custer Drive
Lexington
KY 40517-4001
USA
Website: http://lexington-on-line.com/naf.html

National Center for Post Traumatic Stress Disorder (USA)
Website: http://www.ncptsd.org/

Depression and Bipolar Support Alliance
730 N Franklin Street, Suite 501
Chicago, IL 60610-7204
USA
Tel: 1 800 826 3652
Fax: 1 312 642 7243
Website: http://www.ndmda.org

National Institute of Mental Health
6001 Executive Blvd, Room 8184, MSC 9663
Bethesda MD 20892-9663, USA
Tel: 1 301 443 4513
Website: http://www.nimh.nih.gov

National Mental Health Association (NMHA)
2001 N Beauregard Street, 12th Floor
Alexandra, VA 22311
USA
Tel: 1 703 884 7722
Fax: 1 703 684 5968
Website: http://www.nmha.org

No Panic
93 Brands Farm Way

Telford
Shropshire
TF3 2JQ, UK
Tel: 0808 808 0545 (helpline 10am–10pm daily)
Website: www.no-panic.co.uk

Obsessive-Compulsive Foundation

337 Notch Hill Road
North Branford
CT 06471, USA
Tel: 1 203 315 2190
Fax: 1 203 315 2196
Website: http://www.ocfoundation.org

Royal College of Psychiatrists

17 Belgrave Square
London SW1X 8PG, UK
Tel: +44 (0)20 7235 2351
Fax: +44 (0)20 7245 1231
Website: http://www.rcpsych.ac.uk/index.htm

SANE

1st Floor
Cityside House
40 Adler Street
London E1 1EE, UK
Tel: +44 (0)20 7375 1002
Freephone: 0845 767 8000
Fax: +44 (0)20 7375 2162
Website: http://www.sane.org.uk/

Triumph over Phobia

PO Box 1831
Bath
BA2 4YW, UK
Tel: +44 (0)1225 330353
Website: http://www.triumphoverphobia.com

Index

Page numbers followed by 'f' indicate figures: page numbers followed by 't' indicate tables.

This index is in letter-by-letter order, whereby spaces and hyphens in main entries are excluded from the alphabetization process.

Abbreviations used in the index are given on page vi

Cross-references are assumed between proprietary drug names and their generic name